COVIDIANS & COVIDOLOGY

COVIDIANS & COVIDOLOGY

Facts, common sense, and simple
science you can understand

(Not recommended for conspiracy
theorists and Trumpians)

Dr. Yasser Negm

ISBN: 9798695296211

Printed in the United States of America

Translations: Amgad Abouamasha & Yasser Negm
Interior designer: Adina Cucicov
Cover designer: Lauren Johnson

Declaration of conflicts of interest: This book was 100% self-funded. There were no contributions from any parties whatsoever provided for its preparation or production. The author did not and is not receiving any payments from the companies or manufacturers of products mentioned in this book. Any brand names written within the context were included for mere benefit of the readers.

Dedication

To my fellow humans who still have faith
that we are not under the control of evil
hidden superpowers and conspiracies.

To my fellow humans who still have
faith that the superpower of mercy and
compassion embraces our world.

To my fellow humans who still have faith
that justice will eventually prevail.

To my fellow humans who still have
faith that the human brain and heart are
trustworthy.

To my fellow humans who still have faith
that science, common sense, reason, and
that the power of people should lead us
to fight and win.

ABOUT THE AUTHOR

Dr. Yasser Negm, an Egyptian-British writer, is a paediatric gastroenterology consultant. He has worked in Egypt, the United Kingdom, and the United Arab Emirates for more than 25 years. He is a fellow of the Royal College of Paediatrics and Child Health (RCPCH) in London and member of the European Society of Pediatric Gastroenterology, Hepatology, and Nutrition (ESPGHAN).

He has penned various writings that include his visions and views on public affairs. He has no affiliation to any organizations or currents of any type except medical professional societies.

You can check Dr. Yasser Negm's curriculum vitae on LinkedIn:
https://www.linkedin.com/in/yasser-negm-967135145/.

He has a website (yassernegm.com) for his writings in Arabic, which contains more than 500 articles, stories, reports, audios, and videos.

His Facebook page (https://www.facebook.com/Dr.Yasser.
Negm/) has more than 129,000 followers.

THIS BOOK

In these uncertain times engulfed by clouds of doubts, suspicion, panic, lack of scientific and logical thinking, and inability to plan even for the near future, I have opted, as a physician, researcher, and writer within the human community, to decipher some haunting mysteries, de-obscure the overall foggy situation, and disengage the alleged conflict between science and quackery.

We are not yet aware of many details about that "novel" unknown organism which has taken our world aback, threatened human life, and turned it upside down. Although we are still in the "crawling" stage to come at grips with the virus, we have a thousand-year repertoire of common sense, hundreds of years of development in preserving public health, and decades of evidence-based medicine.

This book simplifies scientific terminology for the non-specialist reader. It succinctly focuses on straightforward practical information: no profuse introductions, no enigmatic theories, and no boring details that may repel you, unnecessarily prolong the book, or restrict the required diversity to review all aspects of dealing with the pandemic in everyday life.

In terms of references and sources, I often refer to verified and credible general media sources rather than specialized references. This is to facilitate cross-reference by the reader and go through the same language and terms the general public understand.

As healthcare professionals, we are both debtors and creditors. We owe it to all humankind to guide them in terms of awareness, education, care, treatment, and scientific research during this dreaded pandemic. However, they also owe us to listen to what we say, read what we write, and trust us. They should not surrender their ears, eyes, and minds to the mongers of deceit, addicts to conspiracy theories, idiots of limited intelligence, and advocates of political and commercial agendas that run counter to professionalism, knowledge, honesty, and credibility.

CONTENTS

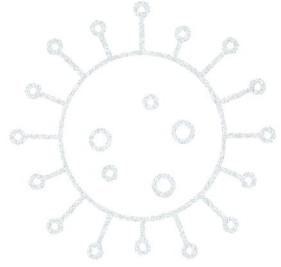

A WORLD IN CHAOS

Save for the rudimentary general information that most people know from the first days of the pandemic, every study that has come up with something new has a counter-study proven the opposite. Each piece of information below has had a study to confirm and another to refute.

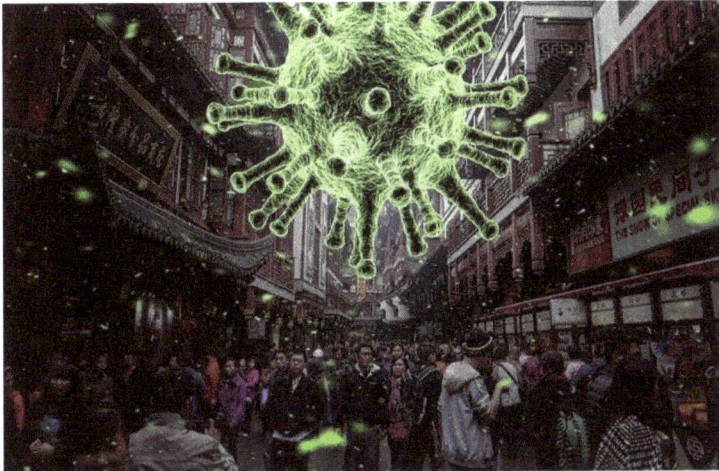

The coronavirus disease is lab-made.	↻	The coronavirus disease has naturally mutated.
The coronavirus disease is airborne transmitted.	↻	Airborne transmission is not possible.
The coronavirus disease spreads easily via contaminated surfaces.	↻	The contaminated surfaces do not cause infection.
Infection can take place within a distance of less than a meter.	↻	You wish! You have it wrong. The coronavirus can travel up to six (6) meters.
Heat kills the coronavirus.	↻	Nope, it does not die because of heat.
Handshaking means infection.	↻	Not at all! This is very wrong.
We must put on facemasks.	↻	This is wrong! Masks are useless.
The coronavirus disease is transmitted via food.	↻	Imposssssssible!
The coronavirus remains contagious for only a fortnight.	↻	Some remained infected for one month and a half.
The coronavirus in China is not the same as in Italy.	↻	No, man! The Italian coronavirus came from China.
The best approach is to let people get herd immunity[1].	↻	Nonsense! The best approach is rather to have the strictest lockdown you can. Otherwise, the death toll will be high!
Tuberculosis-vaccinated peoples are immune to the coronavirus.	↻	This is a fallacy. The coronavirus may kill them as well.

---

1 Also called herd effect, community immunity, population immunity, and social immunity.

The anti-malaria drug kills the coronavirus.	↻	Never. To the contrary, it may rather kill those infected.
The coronavirus disease affects the reproductive organs.	↻	No, it does not.
Reinfection is likely.	↻	What are you saying? Of course not. You will be immune to the coronavirus disease.
The Japanese medicine heals in 4 days.	↻	This is wrong. There is no proof of that because the relevant study is unreliable.
The antibodies test proves you have immunity to the coronavirus.	↻	No, brainiac! The coronavirus disease has mutated into three types any of which can infect you.
AIDS medicines kill the coronavirus.	↻	Nonsense. This is just ta chimera.
The coronavirus affects smokers the most.	↻	No, this is wrong. Rather, smoking may protect against the coronavirus disease.

Let alone the quackery of gurgling with vinegar and lemon and the charlatanism of the 5G and conspiracy theory addicts. I only refer to scientific studies. The above self-contradictory claims are part of scientific research published by prestigious entities. Thus, the public is not blamable after their lives have turned upside down out of the sudden rendering them in dire need for any information regardless of its source. How about information from allegedly well-documented scientific studies!

The blame is on the chaotic publishing. This applies to scientific publishing in reputable medical journals. Many researchers wanted to gain even if at the expense of the recognized quality standards. It also applies to the media outlets, which have become, regrettably, kiosks for the statements of this or that professor or research. The average person, and even the average physician, cannot differentiate between the scientific studies in terms of quality, weight, and credibility to separate the wheat from the chaff.

Well. I can hear somebody saying: You keep on advising us to follow science not myths and conspiracies, while you are admitting that science has failed to provide answers!!!

Here, comes the role of evidence-based practice.

Evidence-based medicine, where specialists read books and receive trainings and courses, has only one purpose, namely to differentiate between the reliable and deplorable scientific studies whose only place is the dustbin of history though dubbed "scientific" and issued by reputed scientific bodies. Even a university professor who has not received training in evidence-based medicine should not judge such studies.

In the past, people used to dub inefficient the physician who does not keep pace with scientific studies. However, this has changed 15-20 years ago, as the inefficient physician has become the one who applies what he reads or listens to in a conference. The excellent specialized physician does not apply all that they hear or read but rather the highest grade of evidence issued in the form of treatment protocols agreed upon by the specialized scientific bodies to avoid the suspicions of personal interests and lack of high quality standards.

What at stake here is that the perpetuation of this chaos will make people lose confidence in science altogether because for every advice or consultancy a physician or a scientist would provide, a swindler may provide the opposite based on a study as well. Then, the quackery-based option and the scientific option will be equal as along as science, presumably though, says both options are acceptable.

This book as well as similar publications by my honest, competent colleagues are part of these efforts to clear the smoky fog. Let's explore together the accounts of Covidians; patients, families and professionals who encountered the monster and Covidology; highly evidenced science of the epidemic.

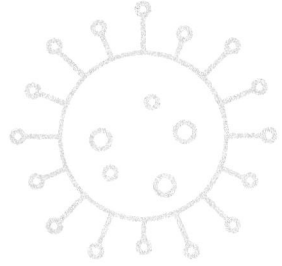

CHAPTER 1

FROM THE MEMORY OF HUMAN RACE: THE SPANISH FLU IN PHOTOS (1918–1920)

(source: US national archives)

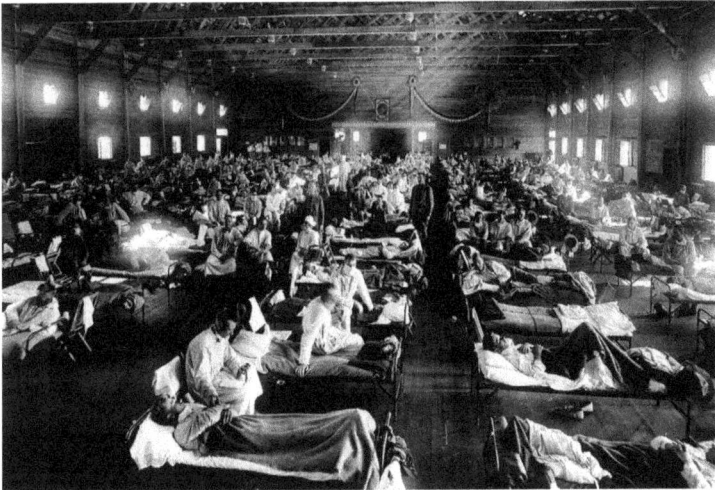

Emergency flu hospital—Kansas—USA

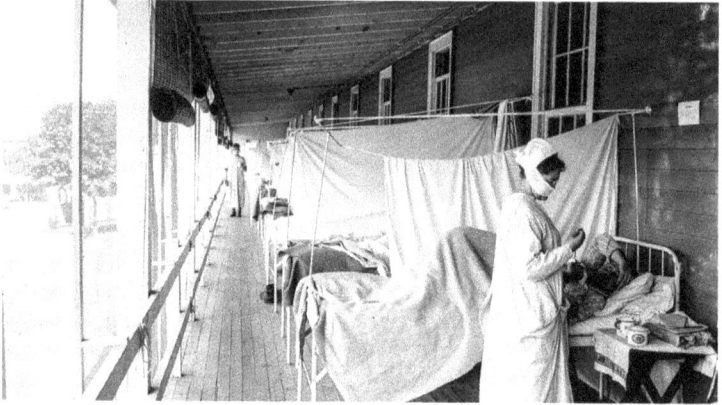

Healthcare concepts at the time recommended care for flu patients in open air . Walter Reed, the same hospital where Donald Trump was treated for Covid 19 in October 2020

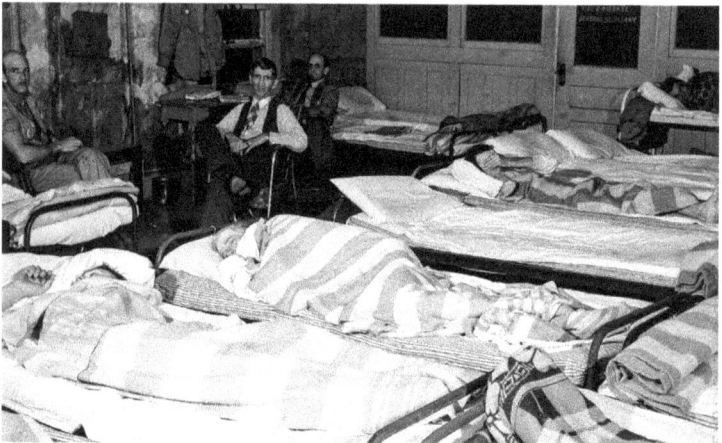

Flophouses overcrowded with low income workers were major contributors to spread of flu100 years ago, and still for Covid 19 today

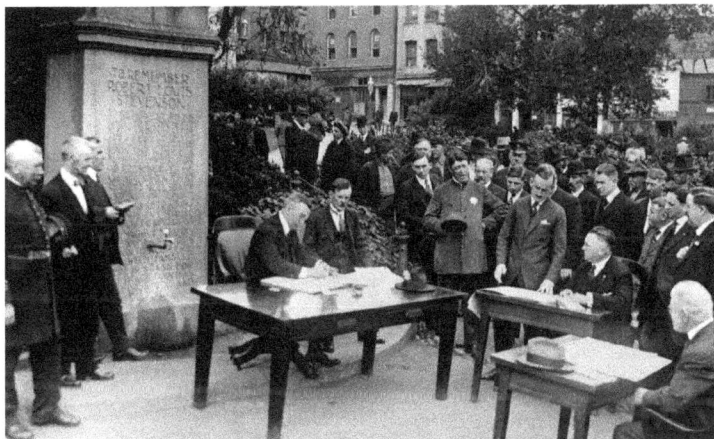

Court proceedings held in open air.
It was mandatory for all events to be run in open air
according to healthcare concepts at the time

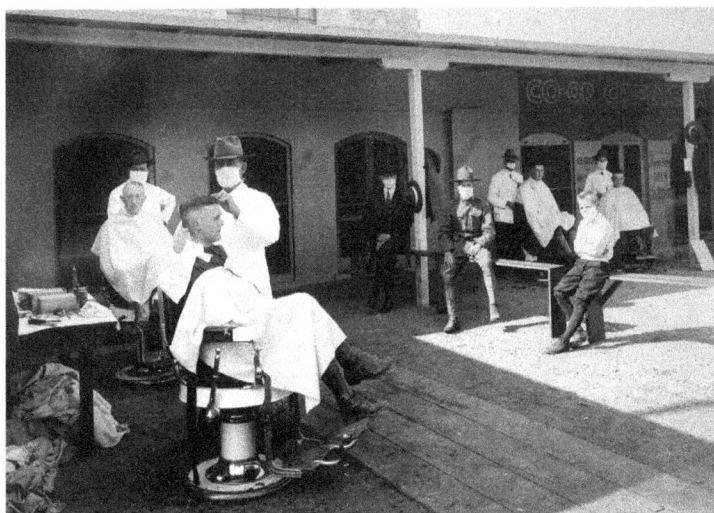

Haircut in open air

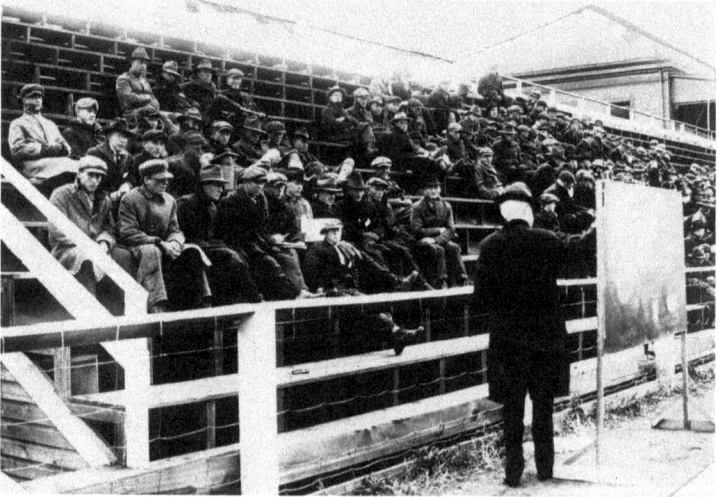

University lecture in open air

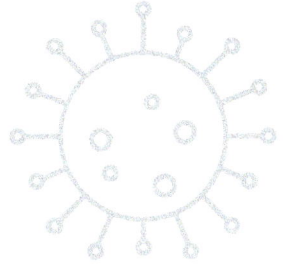

CHAPTER 2

RETURN OF THE AVENGER: A GLIMPSE OF CORONAVIRUS HISTORY

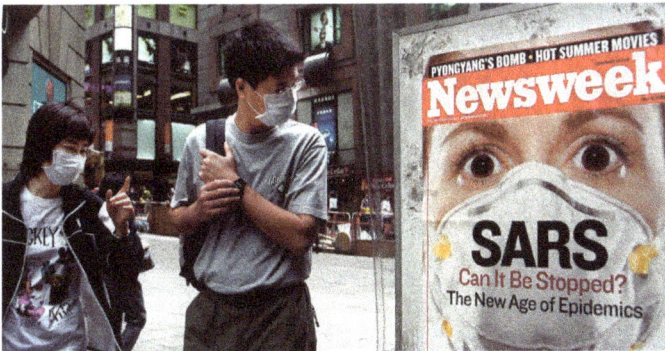

Hong Kong—May 2003

Its official scientific name is: severe acute respiratory syndrome coronavirus 2 (SARS-CoV-2). We all know it now as it has turned our world upside down and brought the plans of 7.8 billion people to a standstill. It came from nowhere to kill, destroy and damage.

But, wait for a minute. Did it really come from nowhere? Conspiracy theorists might have been right then!!!

Nope. Absolutely not.

Coronavirus2 is the descendant of a famous gang of serial killers, the coronavirus family which have been known to us at least for half a century. The novel descendant is exactly the seventh descendant of the family. The family are categorized as "zoonotics"; meant to live only inside animals not humans. Yet, they have been relentlessly and repeatedly attempting to invade us.

The 16th of November 2002 marked the first success of its kind for the coronavirus family to infect human beings, kickstarting the first epidemic of the 21st century in Foshan, China; the SARS epidemic.

The SARS epidemic was quite voracious for human lives, with a death rate of 10% (3 times the current rate of Covid 19) and R0[2] of 3 (Every case transmitted infection to 3 other people on average). In spite of that, the number of lives claimed by that epidemic was quite limited if compared to Covid 19 (total of approximately 8000 deaths in

---

2   Ro is the expected number of cases directly generated by one case in a population where all individuals are susceptible to infection.

9 months). By July 2003, the epidemic was over; thanks to the efficient outstanding response of the government of china at the time, and surrounding countries with support of the World Health Organization (WHO). Comparing such case with the current Covid 19 situation, the Chinese government and also WHO deserved the heavy criticism they received for delayed incompetent responses and lack of transparency which accumulated a mount of more than 50,000 cases in China alone between end of December 2019 and mid-February 2020.

The coronavirus had to mutate[3] to be able as a zoonotic to invade human beings during the 2003 SARS epidemic. Yet, after its defeat, it had to mutate again for a comeback.

The comeback occurred in 2012 with the emergence of another epidemic: MERS; Middle East Respiratory syndrome. It appeared first in Saudi Arabia, Qatar and Tunisia. It was a very slowly spreading epidemic; affected roughly 1000 persons in lazy waves over an extended period of 6 years. We should be thankful to such character, as the MERS epidemic had a really scary death rate of 30%. Had the current novel coronavirus been such lethal, we

---

3   It is the change of genetic information passed to the next generation, acquiring new characters probably in favor of the viral ability to survive and invade

would have been mourning more than 10 million souls in the past few months.

The family's revenge for SARS and MERS appeared in an unregulated raw food market, Wuhan, China, December (possibly November) 2020. The new thug arrived armed with spikes covering 2 layers of fat. It imitated a family friend (HIV) for a top weapon: Furinase, an enzyme which multiply its attachment power to human membranes by 10 times. This is exactly what it needed to challenge 7000 years of human civilization, 700 years of scientific progress and 70 years of modern welfare.

⚙ COVIDIOLA FROM YESTERDAY

- The Spanish flu did not emerge from Spain
- Spain was not the country most hit by the epidemic
- It was the neutral Spanish media, free from censorship providing the world with the most comprehensive coverage of its news which gave the epidemic this name.

References: 1—5

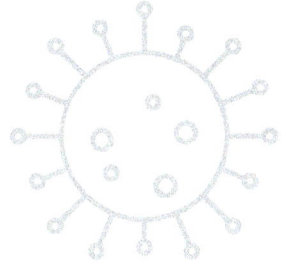

CHAPTER 3

GOOD VS BAD SCIENCE & SOURCES OF RELIABLE INFORMATION

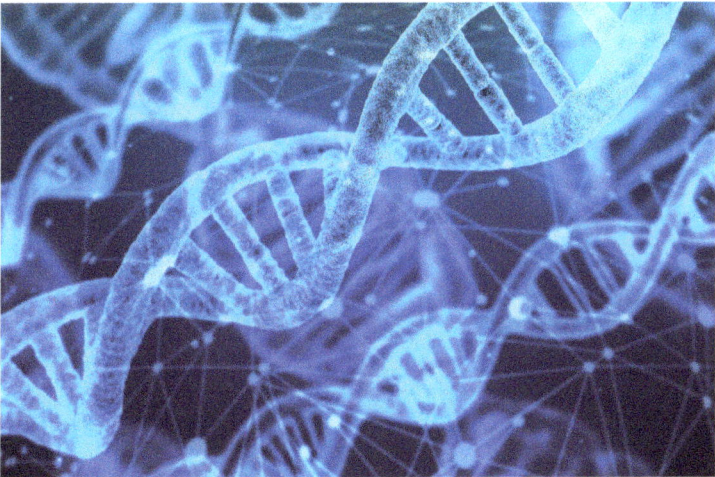

The majority of us nowadays google health updates, news, seeking a treatment or specialists' recommendations in relation to nutritional, natural or medical products, diseases like Covid and its treatments, advances or medical equipment. You may receive information also over social media or hear something from a family member, friend or neighbor. You may watch a youtuber or a blogger brainwashing her audience on how fantastic or how awful this experience or that. You might be a fan of homeopathy and websites advocating natural remedies.

I have a duty to tell you that all of this have never been a subject of scientific validation. What benefits somebody pose a risk to another and vice versa. Science has its extremely reliable way of testing to explore the good and bad for every one by robustly experimenting on huge numbers of people under strict neutral conditions.

The scientific progress over the past 50 years did not only embrace development and innovation of content. More importantly it comprised robust quality assurance of the methods this scientific content has been practiced and whether the outcomes are conscientiously and accurately sound. Like all other fields of professions, quality guarantee systems have been overwhelmingly of utmost importance to make sure the advances are competent with the current and future levels of human welfare. In healthcare, this concept has become even more complex due to its nature guarding the safety and wellbeing of people. If wrong estimates, personal interests and bias are allowed into Medicine, the cost would be millions of lives, no civilized community can afford such price.

In brief, what we call "Evidence Based Medicine" has a hierarchy. Single expert opinion is at the base of this hierarchy, while a consensus of such experts ranks higher.

An unpublished study which hasn't been reviewed by a peer in the field is out of the window, better in the dustbin.

A study of a medicine in the lab with some good results, but hasn't been tried on humans could be promising, but still not a sound scientific evidence.

A study on a huge number of patients already peer reviewed and published in a well-recognized journal mounts to a good evidence but still not the best.

If the study includes observations over a period of time is better.

A clinical trial comparing the medicine to another with neutralization of all biasing factors is stronger.

If we can blind the practitioners and the researchers, so that they do not know which medicine was tried on which patients, this ranks very high (Double blind randomized controlled trial).

When the evidence from such study outweighs similar studies as per experts' systematic review, then we have achieved the strongest possible evidence. This is good science.

Yet, still the world is not that ideal and rosy in the field.

Certainly you cannot look for the evidence and its strength yourself. Most doctors can not as well, either because they are not trained to do it or due to the inability to follow all the new evidence. The number of medical studies published in well-recognized journal exceeds 125000 articles annually. Every 5 minutes, a new article is published in a well-recognized journal, let alone the more abundant second and third degree journals in addition to pseudoscience journals. By the time we sleep at night and wake up next morning, 100 new articles would have been published.

Is it all good science?

Definitely not. If we are optimistic, 85% would be bad science. What is applicable to our everyday healthcare is a minority of the 15% good science.

Most of what you find in google, receive on social media, read in the news, and hear from friends and family is either bad science, pseudoscience or no science at all. We have not discussed yet the dubious funding of research by pharmaceutical companies (directly and indirectly) to twist the research serving their own interests.

Some of the study results you encounter in general media are there only, because the researchers have good connections with the media or due to their positions in authoritative bodies. Frequently, it has not anything to do with credibility of the research.

What should we do then?

Internet wise, you should only rely on a handful of trust-worthy resources, which are very unlikely to be biased by financial interests, trends, ideology or unqualified admin-istrators. Usually websites of scientific societies, patient groups and charity organizations are duly respectable in that aspect.

Practice wise, your trusted doctor is the best to consult. A doctor who listens and talks to you long enough to find out whether she is honest, clever, qualified and up to date. Whether your doctor is going to refer you or treat you himself, he will be able to follow you up and show adequate care and empathy. Doctors of this quality belong to highly specialized medical societies which review and update the strongest evidence regularly and update all members with the top guidelines and protocols.

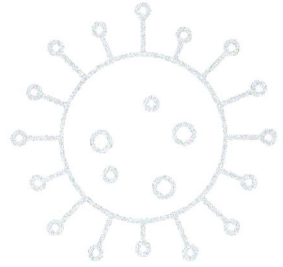

CHAPTER 4

MARCH OF THE VIRUS

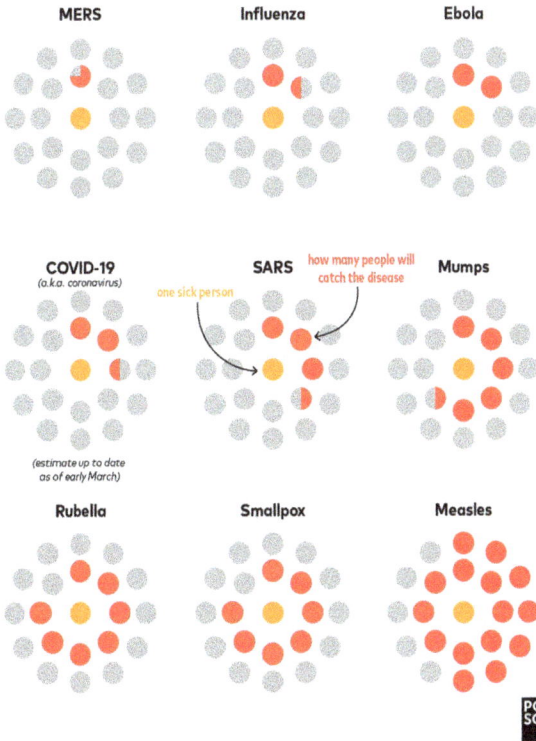

MERS

Influenza

Ebola

COVID-19
(a.k.a. coronavirus)

SARS

one sick person

how many people will catch the disease

Mumps

(estimate up to date as of early March)

Rubella

Smallpox

Measles

POP SCI

This chart compares the R0 of different viruses. R0 is the number of contacts contracting infection from the original case on average. So, it is a measure of the power of the virus to infect. In other words, it reflects how fast and broad the virus can spread. As you can see, the measles is the worst (Thanks to vaccination saving millions every year). The laziest is the MERS (Fortunate as well because it is very deadly with a mortality rate of 30%).

Covid 19 or in more scientific term: SARS-COV-2 stands as average. Its R0 is 2.5; each case transmits the infection to 2-3 contacts in average. It is comparable to Ebola, less infective than SARS and more infective than seasonal flu.

The main route for transmission of infection for Covid 19 (like other respiratory infections) is direct contact (less than 1.5 meters distance) with a coughing or sneezing carrier of the virus. Also, loud speaking of the infected person can spread the infection to people in close contact. The possibility of transmission is directly proportional to the duration of contact. More details on this issue will come up in later chapters. Whether the transmission is airborne or not is still debatable.

An interesting story related to that has been published in "Emerging infectious diseases", the official journal of the Chinese centers for disease control and prevention:

Mid-April 2020, a stroke patient at a local hospital in the Chinese province of Heilongjiang was diagnosed to have covid19. This was surprising, as the area was declared Covid free on the 11th of March. Two sons of the patient were found to test positive as well.

A comprehensive screening was done for all the hospital patients and staff. Twenty (20) other people tested positive, but it did not stop there. This patient has been to another hospital previous to admission to this hospital, between the 2nd and the 6th of April. When tested, 28 more people were Covid 19 positive. The stroke patient has attended a party before falling sick, specifically on the 29th of March. Swabs were done for all guests of the party. 19 were infected. Among the guests, a lady and her friend visited earlier the lady's daughter 10 days before the party. This daughter also caught the infection.

On reviewing the information of the residents where the daughter lives, it was discovered that one of the residents returned from USA the same day the lady visited her daughter.

The traveler lives one level above the daughter. The traveler had no symptoms at all and tested negative on airport swab. This was a dilemma. To confuse the investigators more, she was found to be adhering to the quarantine rules very strictly. The team was shocked by the result of antibody testing of the traveler. The antibodies were quite high. She had it then!!!!

In spite of being asymptomatic??!! Yep

In spite of test negativity??!! Yep

Based on the fact that the traveler never mixed with her neighbor, nor her neighbor's mother or friend, it was concluded that the transmission of infection occurred indirectly through the building lift, which was used by the traveler shortly before her neighbor's family. From there, the virus marched steadily and heavily to invade 68 other people in an area which was covid19 free prior to this incident.

☼ COVIDIOLA FROM YESTERDAY

Meticulous studies including detailed genetic analysis of the COVID virus have undoubtedly proven that it is not man made and not a lab product.

It is the development of natural mutation.

The strongest evidence of such conclusion came in March 2020 from Nature, one of the top scientific journals in the world. The authors included leading experts in the field from USA, UK & Australia

Who would have done it?

- Can't be China: It hit most Wuhan, the heart of Chinese industry
- Can't be USA: Trump himself has got it
- Can't be anybody else: No human being in the world is safe from catching it himself or his beloved ones

References: 6, 7, 12

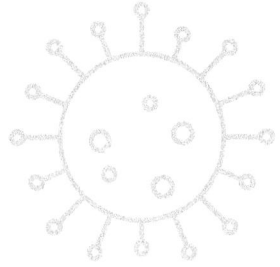

CHAPTER 5

COUGHING AND SNEEZING ETIQUETTE

Despite the outbreak of the novel coronavirus pandemic throughout the world, many people do not know the etiquette of coughing and sneezing. All people need to spread health awareness to preserve their safety and that of their loved ones and the entire society:

- Cough or sneeze into your sleeve or the crook of your arm.
- Sneeze in a disposable tissue rather than a handkerchief.
- Turn away from people when coughing or sneezing so as not to infect others.
- Always wash your hands with soap and water for at least 20 seconds several times a day.

COUGH ETIQUETTE

Cough into your sleeve or the crook of your arm. Coughing into your hand spreads germs.

Cough into a handkerchief or a tissue. A tissue is better because it is disposable.

Turn away from people when coughing. Germs can spread through airborne droplets.

Always wash your hands with soap and water. This prevents the spread of germs.

FAST FACTS

20 seconds
The amount of time it should take to wash your hands.

6 metres
The distance droplets from a cough can travel.

1 in 5
The number of people who do not wash their hands.

SOURCES:
https://www.health24.com/Medical/Cough/News/how-far-can-a-cough-travel-20171207
https://www.cdc.gov/handwashing/when-how-handwashing.html
https://www.sciencefocus.com/the-human-body/how-far-do-coughs-and-sneezes-travel/

health24

- The infectious droplets can travel up to six (6) meters (as a general rule for the easily spreading respiratory bugs, not specifically coronavirus).

COVIDIOLA OF TODAY

Covid19 virus does not spread from animals, does not spread from food, may spread by shaking hands,and may spread through touching surfaces recently contaminated by infected body secretions.

References 8,9

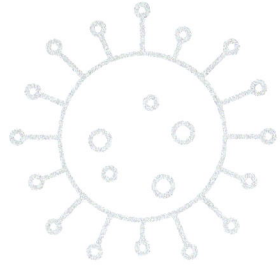

CHAPTER 6

DESTROY IT OUTSIDE YOUR BORDERS

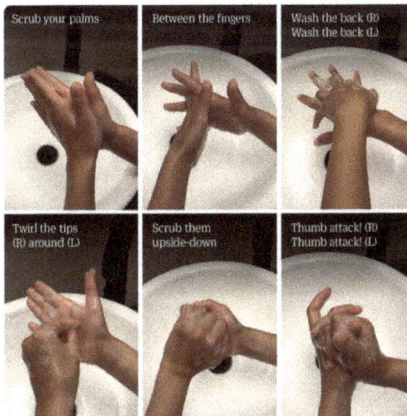

| Scrub your palms | Between the fingers | Wash the back (R) / Wash the back (L) |
| Twirl the tips (R) around (L) | Scrub them upside-down | Thumb attack! (R) / Thumb attack! (L) |

Once the virus (any virus) entered your body, there is nothing voluntary you can do. It is out of your hands. The fight will start between your defense immune system and the invading forces. The outcome of this war depends on the strength of your immune system at the time and the quantity and strength of the infection.

Ideally, you should avoid this war, destroying the enemy while it is still outside your borders.

The clues to this include: social distancing, masks (will be discussed in later chapters), hand washing and sanitization.

The picture shows the proper technique of hand washing which should continue at least for 20 seconds, preferably for 40 seconds and 1 whole minute for healthcare workers. Fortunately, water and soap are adequate to get rid of most bugs including the coronavirus, either by killing them or at least washing them away.

Hand sanitization using ethyl alcohol 60-70% is even more effective in killing 99.9% of bugs including coronavirus. Beware not to use alcohol less than 60% as it not as efficient, ant not to use methyl alcohol (methanol) as it is toxic and not suitable for hand sanitization.

Chlorinated water with a concentration of 1 : 50 (chlorine : water respectively) is powerful for cleaning surfaces.

_____

Reference 10

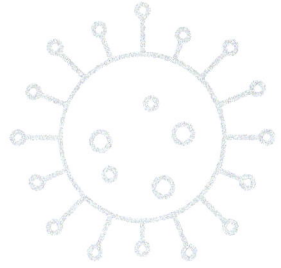

CHAPTER 7

IMPACT OF SOCIAL DISTANCING ON THE PANDEMIC

Free-for-all

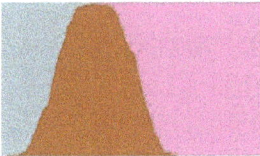

Attempted quarantine

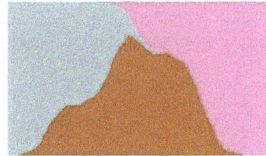

Moderate distancing

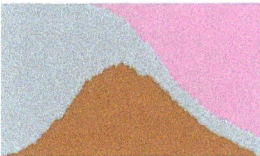

Extensive distancing

The above four pictures show four different outbreak situations of the pandemic.

Up left: Do Nothing

In this case, though the virus will not last for long, it will spread like wildfire killing tens of millions within months and then end. This what used to happen in old ages.

Up right: Infected Cities Quarantined

In this case, the virus will remain for a relatively long time, but it will claim the lives of fewer people mostly inside the quarantined cities. This what china did in Wuhan at a later stage.

Down left: Moderate Social Distancing

Moderate social distancing throughout the country even in the areas with low rate of outbreak. Make people take leaves, close socializing places, make them hate to go out, and shut off any outdoor entertainments. In this case, the virus will last even longer, but it will kill limited number if applied before it is too late. This what most countries did with the current epidemic.

Down right: Complete Curfew

This is the quickest way to get rid of the pandemic with the least death toll provided its timely application.

We have seen the four cases in different places and times with Covid-19. We have seen the countries that did not do anything and the virus ravaged them, such as Wuhan (initially), Italy, Spain, and Iran. We have seen quarantine on the hotspot regions, such as Wuhan at a later stage, Lombardy, and northern Italy. We have seen social distancing taking place in most countries by closing airports and markets, preventing gatherings, and giving leaves. We have seen the complete curfew in Italy and Iran, and to some extent in Kuwait.

☀ COVIDIOLA OF TODAY

The incubation period for the Covid virus; that is the period between catching the infection and the appearance of symptoms is usually 3-7 days, on average 5 days. The longest proven incubation period was 12 days.

It is estimated that 30% of those who catch the infection do not get symptoms at all, but they can transmit the infection and they develop long term immunity afterwards.

Reference 11, 12

CHAPTER 8

FACE MASKS DO WORK

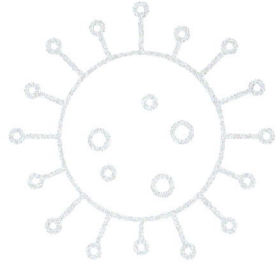

A report published on the CDC (American centers for disease control and prevention) in July 2020 has high-lighted the vital role of masks in halting the spread of infection.

The story took place in Springfield, Missouri—USA, where 2 hairdressers continued to mingle with people for few days, unknowingly they had Covid 19. One of them had symptoms for 5 days, but she continued to work until her test result came out on day 8. She passed the infection to her colleague who started to get the symptoms 3 days later and continued to work until her result came positive a week after. During this period, they dealt directly with 139 customers. Surprisingly, 0 customers caught the infection.

On average, the hairdressers spent 15 minutes with each customer, but they were strict wearing face masks all the time. Also, the customers were compliant with the same. The hair salon as well committed to social distancing rules. The hairdressers would take the masks only during their break time. That's why one of them passed the infection to the other.

A month later, 104 customers were contacted. None of them had symptoms. Only 2 customers took the mask off for some time during their presence in the salon. Nearly half of the customers used surgical masks. The other half used cloth masks. Very few (5% used N95 masks).

Did the hairdressers pass the virus to their families?

One of them passed the infection to 4 members of her family. The other one did not pass it to the 2 people she lives with, as she reported that they do not have that much contact.

Face masks do work.

Please wear them, especially in closed areas and when in vicinity to strangers, as long as this virus is round the corner.

☼ COVIDIOLA OF TODAY

The Chinese rule to protect yourself and your beloved people:

"The key to win against coronavirus is to assume that every person you meet has corona, and to be cautious with every person you meet assuming that you have corona."

Reference: 13

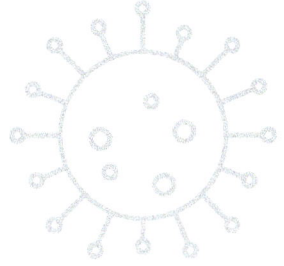

CHAPTER 9

MASKS: TEN QUESTIONS AND ANSWERS

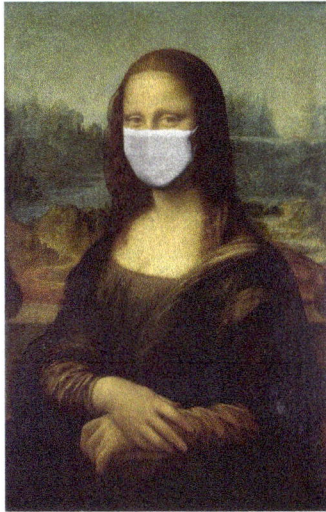

1. **What is the difference between a regular (surgical) medical mask and an N95 mask?**

   The regular mask is not tight around the mouth and nose and thus air can infiltrate whereas the N95 mask/respirator is tight around the mouth and nose so that it does allow such infiltration. It thus filters almost all the air, i.e. ninety-five percent (95%) of airborne particles passing through the mask itself, hence its name "95". As for the letter "N", it stands for "not resistant to oil". It is noteworthy that there are other oil-resistant masks.

2. **What is the benefit of regular medical mask? Does it prevent infection?**

   The regular medical mask isolates the mouth and nose droplets that may be infectious. It also reduces the wearer's touching his nose and mouth with his potentially contaminated hands. However, this mask does not protect against microbial or viral airborne infection.

3. **If the N95 filters ninety-five percent (95%) of the airborne particles, what is the filtering capacity of the regular mask?**

   It filters between ten to ninety percent (10-90%) depending on its quality.

4. **How do we ensure the efficiency of the mask we use?**
   In some countries, there are official authorities responsible for mask quality control. It is better to buy masks with package referring to the approval by such authority in the country of manufacture.

5. **Does the cloth mask help?**
   The size and number of the openings that allow air in the woven cloth mask are much bigger compared to the polypropylene (PP)[4] used in medical non-woven mask rendering it far more efficient.

6. **Would multi-layering of cloth mask improve its efficiency?**
   No. Each additional layer would increase the efficiency by only two percent (2%) and increase discomfort proportionately, which means one cannot put it on for a long time.

---

4   Also known as polypropene, a thermoplastic polymer used in a wide variety of applications.

7. **Is it useful to wear a mask all the time in the current uncertain times?**

Although the World Health Organization (WHO)[5] does not currently recommend wearing it for everyone all the time, some studies have shown that wearing it all the time reduces the infection risk by seventy-five percent (75%). However, the excessive unnecessary purchase of masks will create an availability crisis for those who need them to avoid spreading the infection, such as Covid-19 patients, their contacts, and their treating physicians and nurses.

8. **Is the mask reusable?**

This is not possible for a regular surgical mask. As for N95, it is reusable if not contaminated. However, reusing it makes it more difficult to breathe and increases the chances of microbial growth thereon. As for the cloth mask, wash and reuse.

---

5   Founded on April 7, 1948 and based in Geneva, Switzerland, the World Health Organization is a specialized agency of the United Nations responsible for international public health.

9. **As the WHO does not currently recommend the use of mask for everyone all the time, what does it recommend then?**

The WHO currently recommends the use of masks as follows:

- Not everyone should wear it all the time; social distancing and regular hand washing would suffice.
- Covid-19 patients, those who test positive, and patients of infectious respiratory diseases must wear it all the time.
- Contacts and medical teams treating Covid-19 cases must wear the mask while in close proximity to patients.
- Healthcare professionals must wear N95 when they are very close to patients, such as while installing ventilator tubes.

10. **Some say that wearing a mask may be worse at times than not wearing it. Why is that?**

This is true if the people wearing the masks do not take the necessary precautions in a way that increases the chances of infection:

- If they do not wear and take off the mask correctly.
- If they do not change it when contaminated.

- If they re-use the regular medical mask.
- If they believe that wearing masks replaces social distancing and washing hands.
- If a patient wears it to prevent transmitting the infection to others but does not dispose of it in a hygienic way rendering the mask itself a source of infection.
- If they wear it for self-protection, but touch it from the outside a lot, so the contaminants on the outside of the mask move to their hands.

References 14-16

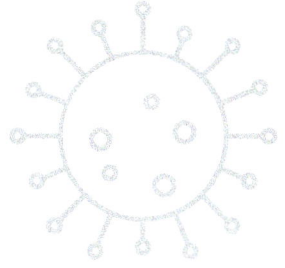

CHAPTER 10

EFFICIENCY RANKING OF 14 TYPES OF MASKS

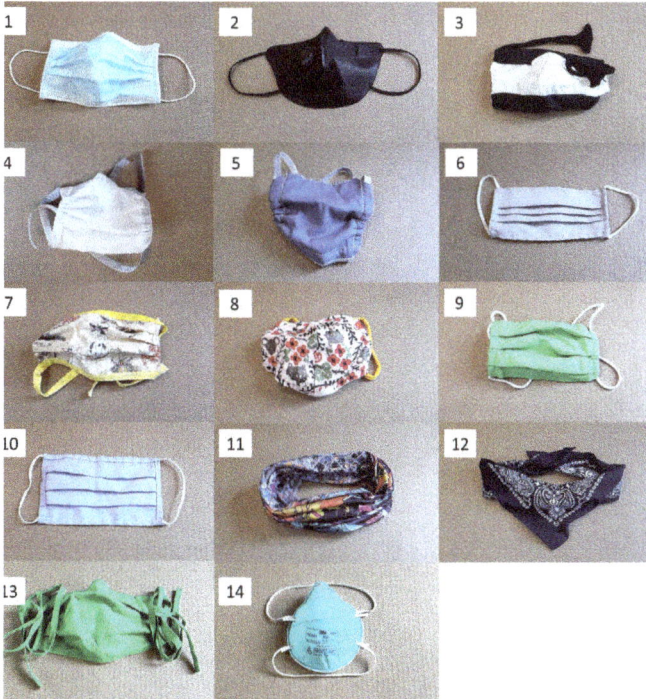

- The most efficient is the fitted N95 (no exhalation valve) (picture 14 above)
- Surgical mask, three-layer (picture 1 above)
- Cotton-polypropylene-cotton mask (picture 5 above)
- Two-layer polypropylene apron mask (picture 4 above)
- Two-layer cotton, pleated-style mask (pictures 7 and 13 above) 2 different types
- N95 mask with exhalation valve (picture 2 above) (Note that the above masks are all more efficient than this mask, which many people do not realize as they think that all N95 masks are the highest in terms of efficiency)
- Homemade two-layer cotton, Olson-style mask (picture 8 above)
- Single-layer Maxima AT mask (picture 6 above)
- Single-layer cotton, pleated-style mask (picture 10 above)
- Two-layer cotton, pleated-style mask (picture 9 above) Different type
- Knitted mask (picture 3 above)
- Double-layer bandana (picture 12 above)
- The least efficient: gaiter-type neck fleece (picture 11 above)

Reference 17

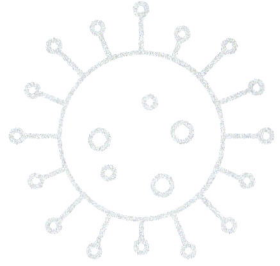

CHAPTER 11

THE USEFUL AND THE USELESS IN PROTECTION

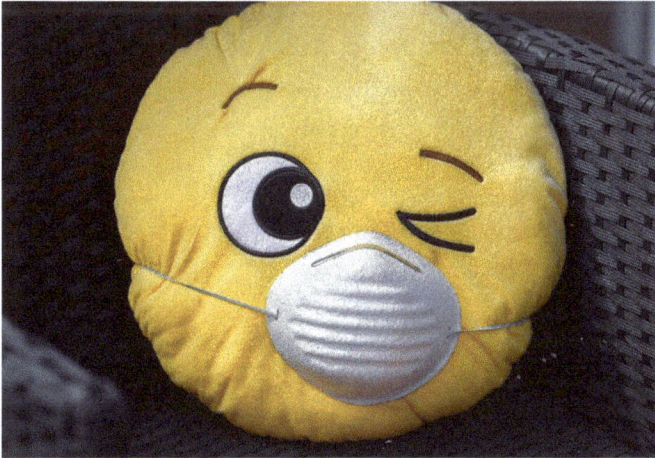

According to scientific evidence,

- **Zinc**: definitely useless and may be harmful.
- **Vitamin C**: often useless but not harmful.
- **Vitamin D**: often useful but may be harmful.
- **Vinegar and lemon gargling**: definitely useless and may be harmful.
- **Hand sanitizer/ disinfectant**: definitely useful and will not be harmful.
- **Azithromycin (Zithromax antibiotic)**: definitely useless and harmful.
- **Malaria medication (Choroquine/Hydroxychloroquine)**: often useless and harmful.
- **Povidone Iodine (Betadine) gargling**: often neither useful nor harmful.
- **Carragelose (Betadine Cold Defense) Nasal Spray**: may be useful and definitely will not be harmful.
- **Social distancing**: definitely useful and will not be harmful.
- **Masks**: definitely useful and definitely will not be harmful.
- **Surface disinfection**: may be useful and definitely will not be harmful.
- **Gloves**: may be useful and may be harmful.
- **Taking off shoes at the door**: neither useful nor harmful.

- **Not shaking hands**: definitely useful and definitely will not be harmful.
- **Enoxaparin (Clexane)**[6]: definitely useless and harmful.
- **Aspirin**: often neither useful nor harmful.
- **Lactoferrin**[7]: often useless and may be harmful.
- **Ivermectin**[8]: definitely useless and may be harmful.
- **Any allegedly preventive diet**: definitely useless and may be harmful.
- **Herbs that boost immune system**: may be useful or harmful.
- **Sleeping well**: definitely useful and will not be harmful.
- **Eating protein**: often useful and not harmful.

---

6 An anticoagulant medication.
7 A multifunctional protein.
8 A medication used to treat many types of parasite infestations.

COVIDIOLA OF TODAY

How to boost your immunity?

The 3 pillars of boosting immunity are not medications, but all natural:

- Good sleep
- Good food
- Good mood

Science has proven that only these 3 pillars are effective in boosting your immune system. Lack of sleep, deficiency of healthy nutrients, mainly proteins, vitamins and minerals with overwhelming junk diet in addition to stress and anxiety suppress your immune responses.

Remember that your natural antibodies which fight infections are made of proteins and that the chemical reactions speeding their function need vitamins and minerals. When you are tired and fatigued from the outside, your body systems suffer the same internally.

Reference 18

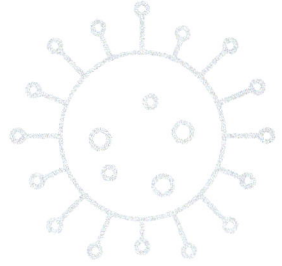

CHAPTER 12

EPIDEMIOLOGISTS AND VIRAL CHASE: A LONG STORY CUT SHORT

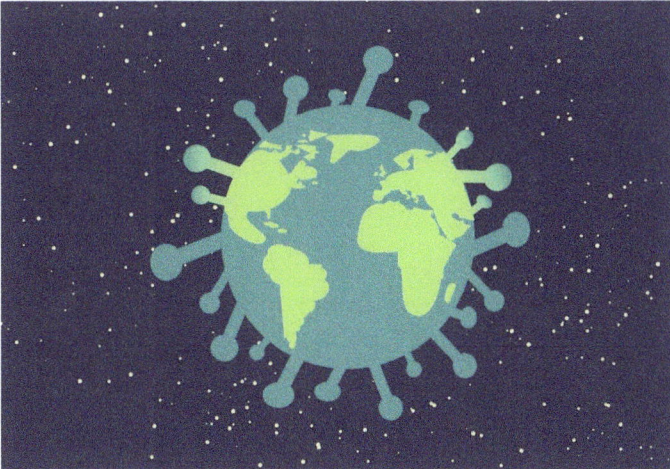

In the following paragraphs, I will address an information that has surprised some friends and raised questions.

It goes that a group of thirty-seven persons contracted the infection on a bus on their way to a worship place. Scientists discovered that thirty-five of them contracted the infection on the bus while only two contracted it in the worship place. How did they know this and determine these numbers accurately?

This is a great opportunity to highlight epidemiology, an obscure discipline to the vast majority of people though it is a vital science for all of humanity in the current circumstances. Of course, this applies to the countries that care about science and benefit from it.

Epidemiologists in such situations work as forensic experts: investigations, evidence collection, and witness testaments. They obtain every important detail in terms of time, place, and surrounding conditions.

In the above situation, they had the seating map of the bus with the seat number of everyone while going and returning. They also checked the seating inside the worship place to check the contacts and symptoms, and when the symptoms, if any, emerged. Of course, if we have the same situation in a subway or a football match in the stadium, the task will be impossible. Here, we have a specific group of people who know one another.

It is very important for the epidemiologists to determine the index case(s)[9], i.e. is the first case(s) that spread the infection. They may find, for example, that all the passengers in the rear third part of the bus contracted the infection while there may be only one or two cases in the remaining parts of the bus. The witness statements may tell them that that case left her seat and headed to the back of the bus to chat with one of her companions for a quarter of an hour during which she transmitted it to her neighbor. In this way, they ascertain that the infection spread on the bus rather than in the worship place. They continue to listen to the statements to find that the back seaters on the bus sat in separate places inside the worship place. They test those who sat beside them. Results came back negative except for two who were not sitting beside them on the bus, i.e. they found out that the infection was contracted inside the worship place. This indicates that the rest of the people who were present and did not come on the same bus might have had a case, but none of the people sitting beside that case contracted the infection.

---

9   The index case or patient zero is the first documented patient in a disease epidemic within a population, or the first documented patient included in an epidemiological study.

Why do they bother and do all this? They could have told all these cases to have home self-quarantine, take medicine, and call the emergency number if they get sick. They exerted that effort to tell us that in terms of transmitting infection, buses are much more dangerous than worship places. Then, when the country lifts the lockdown, it does that based on knowledge and aware-ness and organizes transportation a safe manner, duly follows and controls the spread of the disease and its epicenters, and provides alternative methods that do not spread the disease. At the same time, this country will not deprive its citizens of spiritual or physical needs that would make them happy and comfortable.

There are countries that do not mind to exert relentless efforts and spend their resources on science because they believe this is useful and reflects positively on the future and the welfare of their citizens.

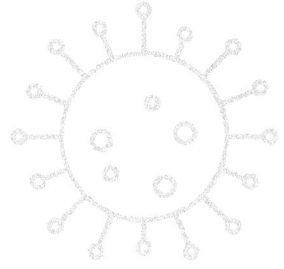

CHAPTER 13

UNDERSTANDING DISEASE PROGRESS: FOR BETTER CONTROL OF THE EPIDEMIC

This picture is extremely enlightening because it at once answers many important questions and refutes many fallacies. First, should someone tell me five months ago that I would use this picture to address the average reader, I would call him crazy. However in 2020, almost everyone has become aware of the latest specialized medical research on a daily basis.

This picture summarizes three respected research papers on the coronavirus published in March 2020 one of which in the Lancet, one of the most renowned medical journals in the world, while the second is the famous Imperial College report submitted to Boris Johnson, the

References:
1. The Incubation Period of Coronavirus Disease 2019 (COVID-19) From Publicly Reported Confirmed Cases: Estimation and Application. Lauer SA et al. Ann Intern Med. 2020 Mar 10.
2. Impact of non-pharmaceutical interventions (NPIs) to reduce COVID19 mortality and healthcare demand. Neil M Ferguson et al. Imperial College COVID-19 Response Team. 16 March 2020.
3. Viral dynamics in mild and severe cases of Covid-19. Yang Liu et al. The Lancet, March 19, 2020.

British Prime Minister, for consideration, and the last in one of the most famous internal medicine journals.

These three abovementioned papers have agreed on the following:

1. There will be no symptoms within the first five days after the patient contracts the virus.
2. Thirty percent (30%) of those who contract the virus develop immunity to the disease immediately after the lapse of the first five days. They feel absolutely nothing and proceed with their lives normally without even knowing they have contracted the virus. However, they remain infectious to others for two weeks. We will revert to this point later.
3. Fifty-five percent (55%) of those who contract the virus will develop mild symptoms for another five days after the first five days. Then, they will proceed in the same way, as the first group does, i.e. no symptoms, developing immunity, and being infectious for two more weeks.
4. After the first five (5) days, ten percent (10%) of those infected will develop severe symptoms that require hospitalization for ten to fourteen (10-14) days. Unfortunately, fifteen percent (15%) of this group, i.e. one point five percent (1.5%) of the total,

die at the end while the remaining eighty five percent (85%), i.e. eight point five percent (8.5%) of the total will live and continue as normal as the above two groups.

5. The condition of the remaining five percent (5%) deteriorates and they enter intensive care. Unfortunately, half of them die, i.e. two point five percent (2.5%) of the total plus one point five percent (1.5%) of the above group, both of which form four percent (4%), the average global mortality. The half that survives proceed like the rest of the groups.

In light of the above, we may conclude as follows:

- The figures of the countries that test only those in intensive care are only five percent (5%) of the real number.
- The figures of the countries that do not test all those in intensive care are lower than that.
- The figures of the countries that test the hospitalized patients who have shortness of breath (SOB) are fifteen percent (15%) of the real number.
- The only reliable figures ate those of the countries that test the ordinary people in the street in hundreds of thousands. Only a few countries in the world do that.

- There are many asymptomatic infectious people. One third of the total cases do not show any symptoms.
- Many people, one third of the total cases, are immune and have never developed symptoms nor taken any test.
- Many people have had a cold for many days, but have never been tested nor diagnosed. They remained contagious for some time while immune (the major ity = more than half of the cases).
- No country will protect its people correctly unless it understands the above and uses it to stem the spread of infection, especially by identifying the infectious persons in the community through more tests.
- No country can test one hundred percent (100%) of its people and thus there is not one hundred percent (100%) control over the virus in any country. However, there is a correlation between the number of tests and the level of healthcare infrastructure on the one hand, and the reduction of death rate on the other hand.
- No country can lift the precautionary measures early and reinvigorate the economy safely unless it understands the above and uses it to identify the community members who have immunity and thus can move freely risk free.

☀ COVIDIOLA FOR TOMORROW

Is re-infection (second infection) possible?

Generally, a person who has been infected by any bug may get a second infection by the same bug. Yet, it should not happen in close intervals in normal conditions, as a person's immune system would have formed antibodies against this particular bug. The presence of these antibodies may continue only for few months, many years or for life.

But there are exceptions: people with weak immunity will have shorter life of these antibodies. Viruses which mutate will deceive the immune system and antibodies will not be able to identify them. Flu virus does that every year. Coronavirus is not an exception to these scientific concepts.

References 19-21

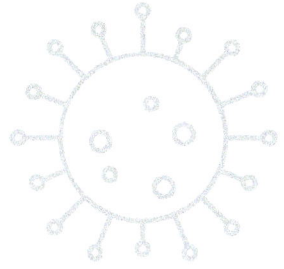

CHAPTER 14

COVID-19 AND CHILDREN:
22 QUESTIONS AND ANSWERS

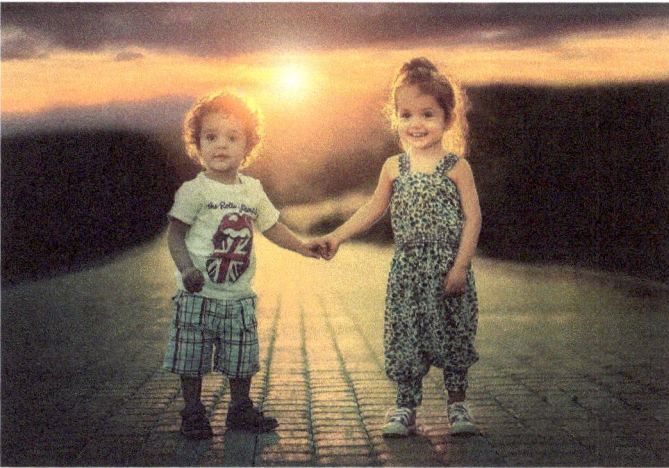

1. **Can children contract the virus?**
   Yes.

2. **Do children transmit the infection to others?**
   Yes.

3. **Do children's symptoms differ from those of adults?**
   They develop the same symptoms.

4. **Does the severity of symptoms in children differ from that of adults?**
   They differ significantly and are much lighter.

5. **Can children develop an infection without showing symptoms?**
   Yes.

6. **Can the situation of children deteriorate like that of adults?**
   Possibly, but this is unlikely. Only six percent (6%) of children need hospitalization and less than one percent (1%) require intensive care.

7. **Is it possible for children to have a cytokine storm[10] in the immune system[11] like adults?**

They develop multi-system inflammatory syndrome (MIS-C)[12]. However, it is rare and treatable in most of them through the intravenous administration of anti-inflammatory and immunomodulatory agents in the hospital.

8. **Does this mean that no children die from Covid-19?**

Very small percentage most of whom have chronic diseases that have weakened their immunity and affected the efficiency of the lungs or the heart.

9. **Do the same isolation rules apply to children?**

Yes, theoretically. However, it is almost impossible to apply this in practice for reasons all of us know. Thus,

---

10 Also called hypercytokinemia. It is a physiological reaction in humans and other animals in which the innate immune system causes an uncontrolled and excessive release of pro-inflammatory signaling molecules called cytokines.

11 The organs and processes of the body that provide resistance to infection and toxins. Organs include the thymus, bone marrow, and lymph nodes.

12 Multisystem inflammatory syndrome in children (MIS-C), also called pediatric multi-system inflammatory syndrome (PMIS or PIMS), is a newly recognized, potentially serious illness in children that seems to be related to COVID-19

we only keep them home to prevent their mingling with children outside the family.

10. **Should children wear masks?**

Only children over six (6) years old.

11. **Are hand sanitizers risky to children?**

No.

12. **Is there a risk to children from touching surfaces frequently outside home?**

There is no need to exaggerate this issue. It is enough to observe social distancing, wear mask, and apply hand sanitizers as much as possible.

13. **Is there a risk from swimming pools and the sea?**

Water itself has no risks but mingling with crowds does.

14. **Is there a risk of group games outside home?**

Yes, if the children mix with a child any of who might be an asymptomatic carrier.

15. **Is there a preventive treatment for children?**

Vitamin D if they have a deficiency. Betadine cold defense nasal spray may be useful.

16. **If symptoms appear, what is the treatment?**

Symptomatic treatment: paracetamol, for example, for fever or pain, cough syrup, medicine for diarrhea, and so on. Vitamin C and zinc may be useful during the episode, not as a protection.

17. **Can we give children antibiotics, aspirin, anti-clotting medicines, or malaria medication at home?**

This is strictly prohibited. These are crimes in the full meaning of the word if given outside hospital setting. This is far more harmful than beneficial.

18. **When should we take the child to the hospital?**

In case of shortness of breath, deterioration in general condition, inability to control the temperature, child's refusal to eat, or the appearance of strange symptoms: spots on the skin, for example.

19. **Can we take a swab from a child? Will the result be accurate?**

Yes, we can. There is no difference in this point between adults and children.

20. **Are there blood tests for children that can tell if they have the virus?**

No, neither for children nor adults but the physician may request tests to diagnose other diseases with similar symptoms or differentiate between bacterial infections that need an antibiotic and viral infections, whether Covid-19 or others.

21. **Is it useful to do a CT[13] scan for children for diagnosis?**

This is another prohibited crime. Exposing a child to unnecessary CT scans dangerously increases the amount of radiation in his body. In case of Covid-19, there is no strong need for CT because there is no confirmation of diagnosis of Covid-19 with any radiation, whether for adults or children.

22. **Does the child take the same time to recover? How long does a child remain infectious?**

Children do not usually fall ill for more than a week. They stop to be infectious after ten (10) days from the onset of symptoms.

---

13 A computerized tomography (CT) scan combines a series of X-ray images taken from different angles around your body and uses computer processing to create cross-sectional images (slices) of the bones, blood vessels and soft tissues inside your body. CT scan images provide more-detailed information than plain X-rays do.

☀️ COVIDIOLA OF TODAY

Why is it more dangerous on the elderly?

It is not only about the weaker body systems, other long term illnesses and deteriorating organs function. There are 3 specific reasons why respiratory infections in general (and not particularly coronavirus) are so dangerous in old age:

- We majorly rely on our chest muscles for breathing. Our body muscles in general get weaker by 2% yearly after the age of 40.
- The elasticity of the small airways get less and less with age. This loss reduces the ability of gas exchange and oxygenation.
- The chest cage gets smaller, decreasing the capacity of the lungs. This happens due to natural kyphosis with age (excessive outward curve of the spine resulting in an abnormal rounding of the upper back).

_____

References: 22-29

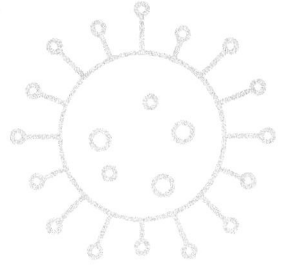

CHAPTER 15

CORONAVIRUS SWAB: IS IT ACCURATE?

The image shows the complexity of the swab test result. In the figure shown, we have one hundred (100) people of whom fifty-seven (57) of them tested positive while forty-three (43) tested negative. However, what is the real situation?

In fact, fifty-six (56) of the fifty-seven (57) already have the virus and one does not. There is a very small percentage of two percent (2%) of people who test positive do actually not have the virus. How do they test positive? Most probably, they have a second virus with a protein similar to that of the coronavirus. However, this is not an important point. The more important is the forty-three (43) who tested negative. These forty-three (43) include twenty-four (24) who have the virus though they tested

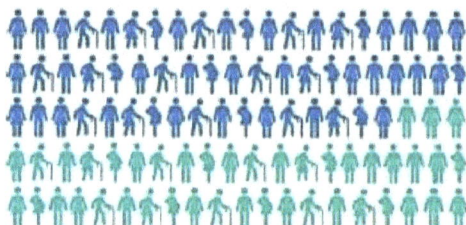

👤 57 people have a test result suggesting that they have covid-19 (test positive)

👤 43 people have a test result suggesting that they do not have covid-19 (test negative)

But who actually has covid-19?

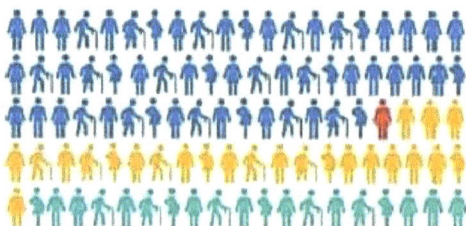

Diagnosis

👤 56 people who test positive have covid-19 ("true positive")

👤 1 person who tests positive does not have covid-19 ("false positive")

👤 24 people who test negative have covid-19 ("false negative")

👤 19 people who test negative do not have covid-19 ("true negative")

Consequences

Appropriately told to self-isolate

Told they need to self-isolate when they would be safe to go out

Told they do not need to self-isolate and so go out and infect more people

Told they do not need to self-isolate and are safe to go out without infecting more people negative. Most of those who test negative, i.e. fifty-six percent (56%) in fact have the virus. However, they test negative, proceed with their life as usual without quarantine, and spread the infection in the community. This is the disaster of the swab test.

What made them test negative?

- The sample was not deep enough.
- The amount of virus was small.
- At the sampling time, the virus did not replicate sufficiently.
- The body's immunity was close to eliminating the virus.

All these are possible reasons. This explains how difficult it is to control this infection despite the quarantine, how a person may die without diagnosis, how a person may contract the infection again, how a person can test negative and then positive, and so on.

Does this then mean that the swab test is useless? No. The swab test remains the most important among all tests and the closest to accuracy. It is much more accurate than blood count, x-ray images, or even relying on symptoms. However, it is better to rely on all of these together. Of course, more accurate tests currently being developed would be more beneficial.

Moreover, the antibodies are more useful in diagnosing a previous infection rather than a new one when it occurs. Until the time we have a more accurate test, it is important to repeat the swab once, twice, and thrice, especially for symptomatic people or those more likely to transmit the infection to a large number of people.

The next chapter reports a breakthrough development of a newer far more accurate and fast test which will be soon universally used.

Reference 30

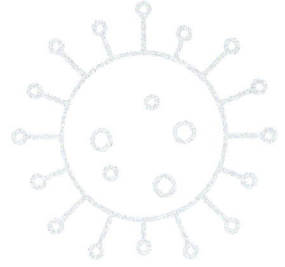

CHAPTER 16

A BREAKTHROUGH: 90%-ACCURATE QUICK TEST

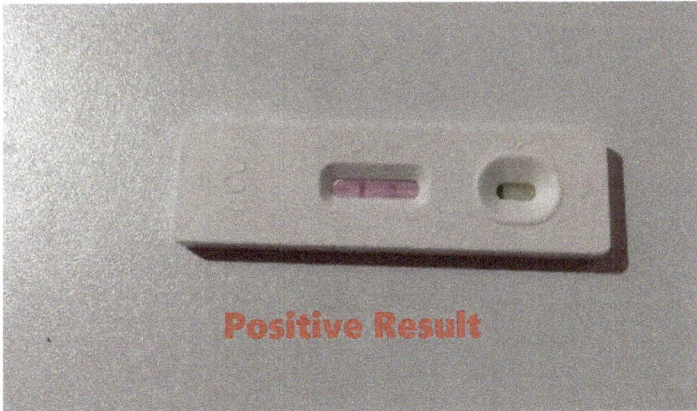

Positive Result

The spread of the Covid-19 pandemic has multiple and complex reasons, one of which is the difficulty of diagnosis due to inaccurate tests and delayed results.

A recent new pivotal shift will greatly facilitate access to accurate and fast diagnosis hence stemming the spread of infection and expediting preventive and curative measures.

The new test, approved officially by the WHO and produced by Abbott Laboratories[14] in cooperation with SD Biosensor Inc.[15] as of September 2020, relies on the nasal swab, but with a ninety percent (90%) accuracy (compared to not more than seventy percent (70%) for previous tests). The result appears within just fifteen (15) minutes in the form of a quick and clear indicator on cards that look like pregnancy test cards.

The cheap price of the new test for poor and developing countries is only US$ 5 supported by the Bill & Melinda Gates Foundation[16] and the WHO is another important positive element.

---

14 Abbott Laboratories is an American multinational medical devices and health care company with headquarters in Abbott Park, Illinois, United States.
15 A South Korean company established in 2010. It operates in the field of manufacturing diagnostic kits.
16 An American private foundation founded by Bill and Melinda Gates. Based in Seattle, Washington, it was launched in 2000 and is reported to be the largest private foundation in the world, holding US$46.8 billion in assets.

The provision of one hundred and twenty (120) million units will take place in the next six (6) months and countries around the world have already started racing to get their share of the test.

References 31

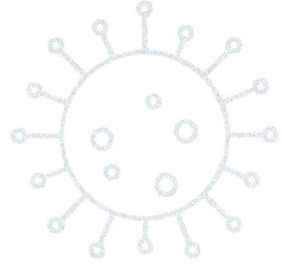

CHAPTER 17

DIAGNOSIS BETWEEN SCIENCE AND NON-SCIENCE

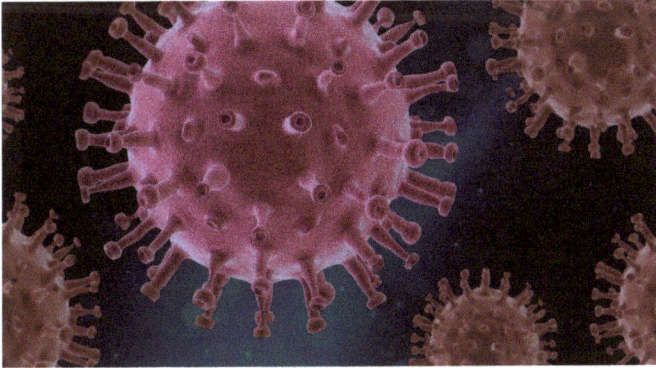

Summary of reliable diagnostic methods for the corona-virus:

- **Blood count**: definitely useless and harmless.
- **D-dimer**: definitely useless and harmless.
- **Ferritin test**: definitely useless and harmless.

- **Erythrocyte sedimentation rate::** definitely useless and harmless.
- **Regular chest x-ray:** often useless and harmless.
- **Chest CT scan:** often useless and definitely harmful.
- **Nasopharyngeal swab (polymerase chain reaction "PCR"):** mostly useful and definitely harmless.
- **Loss of sense of smell and taste:** may be useful in diagnosis.
- **Other symptoms:** cough, fever, diarrhea, and body aches have no value in terms of diagnosis.
- **IgG antibodies in the blood:** have no value in terms of diagnosis.
- **IgM antibodies in the blood:** may help diagnose a recent infection that is not necessarily still present.

Reference 9

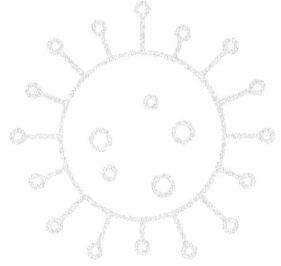

CHAPTER 18

BEWARE OF CT SCAN

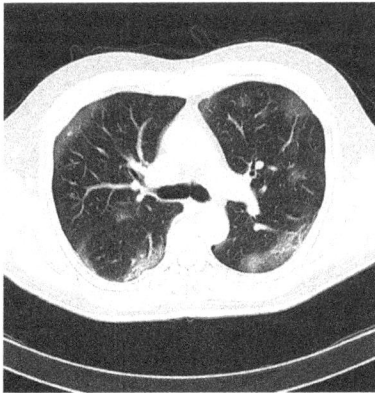

It is my duty as a physician to tell you that a single chest CT has seven (7) millisievert (msv)[17] of radiation compared to only zero point one (0.1) msv for the normal chest x-ray. In other words, one CT scan equals (70) seventy

---

17 The scientific unit of measurement for whole body radiation dose, called "effective dose" named after Rolf M. Sievert (1896–1966), Swedish physicist.

regular x-rays. The one who undergoes one chest CT scan is exposed to (70) seventy regular x-rays, an amount of radiation that the average person is exposed to in two years. If one undergoes three to four CTs, they would equal two to three hundred regular x-ray, equivalent to seven to eight years radiation.

Of course, governments and physicians know this, but ordinary people do not. It is our duty to tell them. I wish people, whether governments, physicians, or patients, do not opt easily to do scans instead of swabbing which is not harmful. Likewise, if a regular x-ray can do, it is better to use it instead of CT.

Of course, if a case deteriorates and enters the intensive care, they will need a CT, but we should not do it for the asymptomatic patient and people with mild or moderate symptoms, especially that if the case deteriorates, repeated CTs will be necessary.

Do not worry! No one can have cancer due to a single CT scan, but we do not know, especially for young people, if they will need other CTs for other diseases or accidents. It is risky practice to have a scan done every time you are suspected to have the virus, and after a few weeks, you are suspected to have the virus again and thus do it repeatedly unnecessarily. This way, we unwisely increase the risk, let alone if we need it three or four times.

Reference 32 and 33

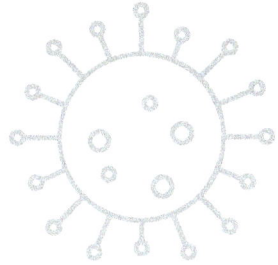

CHAPTER 19

THE STORY OF IMMUNITY, ANTIBODIES, TESTS AND DIAGNOSIS

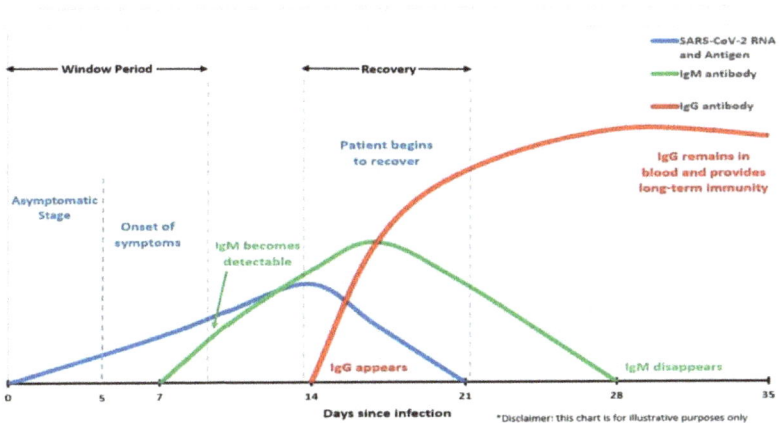

The blue curve represents a positive viral nasal swab. The green curve represents the IgM antibodies, meaning a recent infection, but no diagnosis. This requires a specific blood test. The red curve represents the IgG antibodies (also a blood test), meaning a somewhat old infection and immunity to the virus.

As we see in the picture, the blue swab, which is the only tool for an accurate diagnosis, is positive from the first time one contracts the infection and before symptoms appear up to its acme at the end of the disease. After three weeks of infection, it becomes negative. There are exceptions, but this is the general rule. When the virus subsides, the possibility of transmitting the infection decreases. Some credible studies have indicated it is not infectious after ten to fourteen days.

The green IgM antibodies that the body has produced to resist the virus do not appear until after a week. Thus, the body's resistance in the first days is weak and increases gradually until it reaches its highest level in the middle of the third week.

Two weeks later, the red IgG antibodies start to appear, which coincides with the gradual disappearance of the green ones. The body's highest resistance is at the highest level for both in the third week, which is the time most people get better unless a cytokine storm takes place. After four weeks, only the red IgG remains, with exceptions. These indicate an old previous infection and grant the person long-term immunity to the virus.

Let us wrap up:

- If you doubt that you have contracted an infection in the past few days, but you do not have symptoms, only the swab will be positive if you have actually contracted the infection.
- If you have developed symptoms for the last three to four days, only the swab will be positive, yet again.
- If symptoms persist for the second week, the swab will be positive, but an IgM blood test rather than a useless blood count, ferritin test, D-dimer, and the like, will indicate a recent infection.
- The same applies to the third week.
- If you have had the infection for more than three weeks, you are often no longer infectious, even if the swab is still positive. If you measure the IgG and find it high, you are already immune to the virus.
- If you have recovered for a while and do not know if you have had Covid-19 or another disease and whether you have immunity or not, do an IgG test.

Reference 9

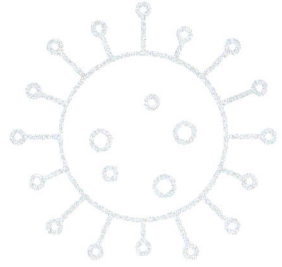

CHAPTER 20

HOW DO YOU DEAL WITH THE CORONAVIRUS DISEASE?

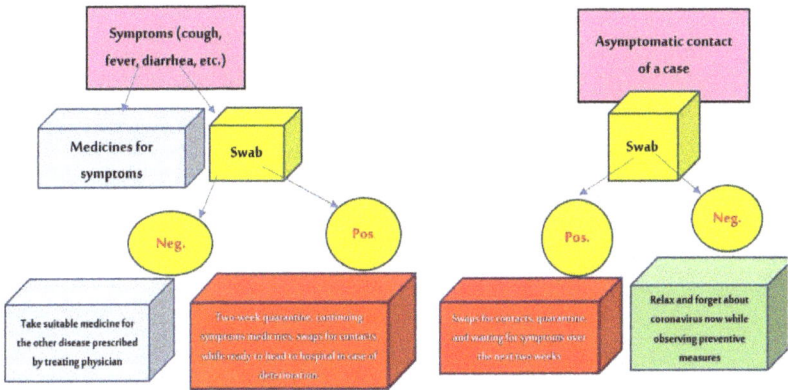

Medicines safe for all patients include: paracetamol for fever, herbal and natural medicines for cough, Kaolin, Pectin and Racecadotril for diarrhea.

Medicines useless with coronavirus include Tamiflu, Metronidazole, Nefuroxazide, antibiotics, and multivitamins.

Medicines not to be taken without a prescription include aspirin, Hydroxychloroquine, Azithromycin, and Salbutamol and Budesonide nebulizers.

Medicines which may help and will not cause harm include vitamin C, vitamin D, and zinc.

If you start feeling shortness of breath and find no place in the hospital, a pulse oximeter for measuring oxygen in blood, a nebulizer, and an oxygen cylinder may help.

Reference 9

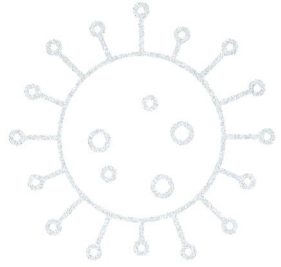

CHAPTER 21

TREATMENT AT HOME AND IN HOSPITAL: EFFECTIVE AND DEFECTIVE

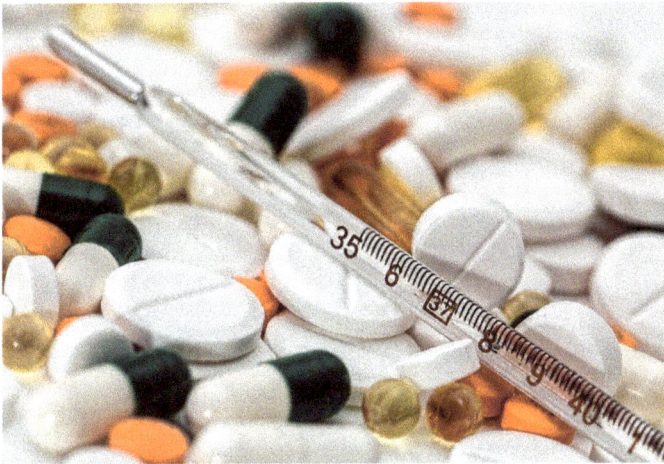

According to the proven scientific findings so far:

At home:

- **Anti-fever and analgesics**: definitely effective
- **Azithromycin**: often defective
- **Other antibiotics**: definitely defective
- **Clexane (Enoxaparin)**: often defective
- **Aspirin**: may be effective under a physician's supervision
- **Zinc**: often effective
- **Vitamin C**: may be effective
- **Tamiflu**: definitely defective
- **Vitamin D**: definitely defective
- **Warm liquids**: often effective
- **Malaria medication (Chloroquine and hydroxy chloroquine)**: often defective
- **Cortisone**: definitely defective
- **Ivermectin**: often defective
- **Lactoferrin**: often neither effective nor defective
- **Cough medicines**: may be effective
- **Celebrex**[18] **(Celecoxib)**: often defective
- **Wormwood, herbs, and fennel flower**: often neither effective nor defective

---

18 It is used to treat the pain and inflammation in osteoarthritis, acute pain in adults, rheumatoid arthritis, ankylosing spondylitis, painful menstruation, and juvenile rheumatoid arthritis.

- **Honey**: often effective
- **Inhaled bronchodilators**: may be effective under a physician's supervision
- **Quarantine/ isolation**: effective and required
- **Pulse oximeter**: definitely effective
- **An oxygen cylinder/ generator**: absolutely effective in case of temporary shortness of breath

In hospital:
- **Cortisone**: definitely effective
- **Inhaled interferon**: often effective
- **Monoclonal antibodies**: Often effective
- **Remdesivir**: often effective
- **Avigan, Russian medicine, and Turkish medicine**: may be effective
- **Malaria medication**: definitely defective
- **Plasma of the recovered**: may be effective
- **Azithromycin**: often defective
- **Antibiotics**: effective in case of secondary bacterial infection
- **Clexane**: often effective
- **Aspirin**: often effective
- **Zinc**: often effective
- **Vitamins**: often effective
- **Tamiflu**: definitely defective
- **Biological treatments**: may be effective

- **AIDS medicines**: often defective
- **Oxygen and respiratory support**: definitely effective

☼ COVIDIOLA OF TODAY

Optimization of home treatment by patients and hospital treatment by doctors is the eventual aim of management. Taking too much which will not work or even can cause harm is as troublesome as neglect of proper treatment.

Reference 9

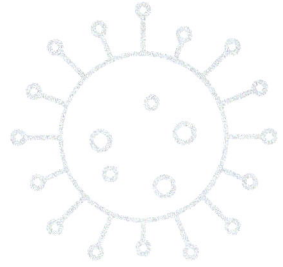

CHAPTER 22

FIRST SUCCESSFUL TREATMENT TO REDUCE THE CORONAVIRUS DEATHS

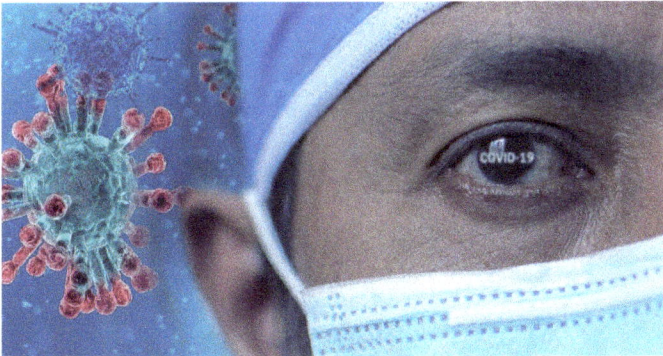

There are three causes for the deaths of Covid-19 patients:

1. A severe infection that causes pneumonia and undermines breathing in people whose immunity is somewhat weak, especially since there is no successful medicine in killing the virus.

2. Elderly patients with several chronic diseases, such as diabetes, cardiomyopathy[19], kidney failure, etc. Severe infection in this case may cause the deterioration of chronic diseases and then death.

3. A patient who has a cytokine storm. Literally, the immune system has gone crazy and started to attack the various body organs and make them fail. It often happens to young and healthy people to some extent. Due to this, since the start of the pandemic, the medical teams used with this last type drugs that inhibit the immune system, including cortisone and biological treatment.

What is new?

A recent scientific study has proven for the first time that dexamethasone, a cheap and available type of cortisone, reduces the mortality rate for critical cases by thirty percent (30%), the last type of deaths. Although it has been part of the treatment protocol for long, the new issue is that a randomized controlled experiment conducted on six thousand (6000) patients has proven that. They administered this medication to a group and administered another drug for another group, which resembles the first in terms of condition, age,

---

19 A disease of the heart muscle that makes it harder for your heart to pump blood to the rest of your body.

gender, other treatments, and everything with the only difference being this medication, and monitored the difference in mortality. They found that the difference is very large, i.e. thirty percent (30%) lower with the Dexamethasone.

Why then cannot we take it at home without a physician's supervision?

First, because if one only has mild symptoms, it will not help. It only helps if one has a cytokine storm.

Second, it inhibits the immune system and thus reduces immunity and allows the virus to prevail.

We want a balanced immune system, neither weak nor insane. We want it 10 out of 10. If it is 20 out of 10, this will cause a cytokine storm; if it is 5 out of 10, the virus will prevail.

Third: The case may deteriorate while not knowing which type. If the case is the type that got worse because the infection has prevailed, dexamethasone will help the virus prevail and may cause death. If it is a cytokine storm, it will help recovery. The physicians at the hospital will know and prescribe the appropriate treatment.

Fourth: The side effects of dexamethasone include hyperglycemia[20], hypertension, nervousness, insomnia, swollen limbs, general weakness, and non-healing of wounds. It may endanger the patients of diabetes, hypertension, stomach ulcers, osteoporosis[21], mental illness, and infection. Thus, never take it on your own. This is a medication that physicians should prescribe in hospitals and it is not an over-the-counter home remedy.

References 34-36

---

20 High levels of sugar, or glucose, in the blood.
21 Loss of bone tissue leading to bone fragility.

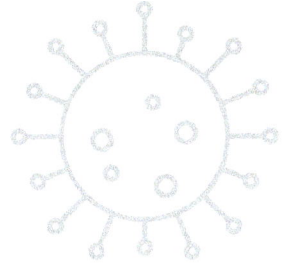

CHAPTER 23

INITIAL SUCCESS OF INHALED INTERFERON WITH COVID-19

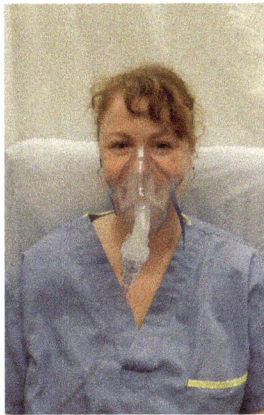

As of July 2020, the interferon beta drug has recorded success in preliminary results of a clinical trial in Britain that involved one hundred and one (101) patients from nine (9) hospitals. The drug has been on the market to treat other diseases.

Tested this time by inhalation, it:

- Reduced the need for respiration by seventy-nine (79%).
- Accelerated recovery from nine to six days.
- Relieved symptom by two to three times faster for the stage of normal activities.
- Reduced difficulty in breathing effectively.

However, the final results are yet to be published.

_____

Reference 37

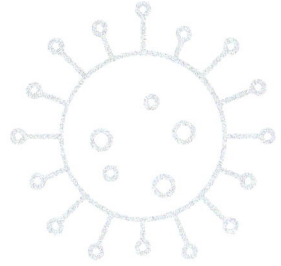

CHAPTER 24

WHY THIS AND NOT THAT? SCIENCE ANSWERS COVID-19 QUESTIONS

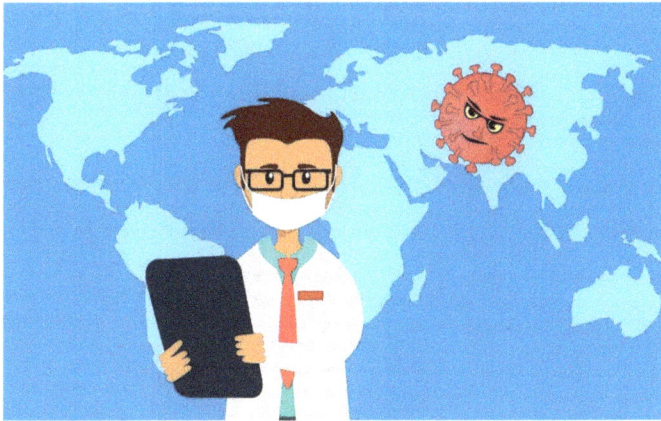

Why is vitamin D good in prevention rather than treatment?

Why are vitamin C and zinc the opposite, i.e. good in treatment and useless in prevention?

Why is taking cortisone at home a bad idea while it is often a success in the hospital?

Why is taking Azithromycin (Zithromax) and Enoxaparin (Clexane) at home "often" not "definitely» a bad idea?

Why aspirin would help if taken under the supervision of a physician and wrong if taken on your own?

Why does malaria medication do more harm than good "often" and not "sure" at home and "sure" in the hospital?

Why are not Ivermectin and Celebrex "often" helpful?

Why is Remdesivir "often" effective while Avigan and its Russian and Turkish versions are the opposite?

Science answers:

- Vitamin D is essential for the immune system because the immune cells need it to function well. However, the question is whether increasing vitamin D in your body above normal would improve immunity. In other words, is it fine to stack vitamin D in your body thinking that the more you take, the stronger your immunity will be? Of course not.

Increasing vitamin D above the normal level will not add any benefit but rather will cause "toxicity", which may lead to vomiting, fatigue, muscle weakness, tissue calcification[22], etc. Therefore, it is useful for your immunity if you have a deficiency and harmful to take if you do not.

If you have a deficiency, how long would vitamin D take to improve immunity? It will take few weeks for its level in blood to be acceptable and then begin to affect the functioning of the immune cells. Thus, if you have a deficiency in Vitamin D, it is good that you take it as prevention so that, within weeks, your immune system benefits and you become ready for the virus. Since most of us have a deficiency, I said that it is "often" useful in prevention.

However, if you has coronavirus, it will not help because if you have a deficiency, it will never have the chance to improve immunity not even in a week or two. If you do not have a deficiency, it will cause vomiting and muscle weakness while already having coronavirus! This is like jumping out of the frying pan into the fire.

---

22 Accumulation of calcium salts in body tissues

- Reliable research on vitamin C and zinc has proven their importance during any respiratory infection. Vitamin C shortens sick days and zinc greatly helps immunity and healing at the time of infection. However, both have no preventive effect. If you do not currently have a respiratory infection, taking zinc and vitamin C will neither improve your immunity nor lead to a prolonged effect if you contract an infection in the future.

- Cortisone is an immunosuppressant with severe side effects, especially if taken for long periods. Since it is an immunosuppressant, it is only useful in calming the disorders of the immune system. If you have a virus without such disorder of the immune system, taking it will strengthen the virus. As regards the coronavirus in particular, it has proven an excellent effect in reducing mortality in critical cases due to the disorders of the immune system.

I hope the picture is clear now: if you take it at home, it will harm you. However, if you are in hospital, the physicians can determine if your type of illness will benefit from that or not.

- Azithromycin is an antibiotic; it does not kill viruses. Some low-level research indicates it can be useful with the virus, but they are not adopted so far and because that, it is "often" useless. As for other antibiotics, no single research, even if weak, says they can be of benefit. Thus, of course, antibiotics in general will "harm" if all people take them in the current pandemic because not only they can not kill the virus, but also massively raise the resistance level of the bacteria in general in the future. The antibiotics will then be like water and will not treat any bacterial infection.

- Clexane prevents strokes; this is its good face. Its ugly face is that if it exceeds a specific limit, it will cause hemorrhage and stroke in hypertension patients. Taking Clexane must be according to a prescription by a physician who knows that the patient has no hypertension or risk of excessive bleeding. The physician should then follow up the condition of the patient through regular blood tests to make sure that there is no bleeding tendency. A very small percentage of coronavirus patients, i.e. one to two percent (1-2%), will have blood clotting all of whom are inpatients in critical condition. Based on the aforementioned, is it useful for us to take it at home on our own? You answer!

- Aspirin helps preventing blood clots, but it is lighter than Clexane in both good and undesirable effects.

- Malaria medication (Chloroquine and hydroxy chloroquine) has been subject to high-level research, but only for hospitalized cases not at home. This research has proven beyond any doubt that its harm is greater than its benefit in these cases. Does it work in mild and moderate cases at homes? We still do not know. However, if we know that ninety-five percent (95%) of the coronavirus cases, whether in the hospital or at home, recover without treatment at all, we should not administer it in hospital and this is even more applicable to home.

- Ivermectin is in a class of medications that treats by killing the worms. They tried it in the laboratory like many medicines with this virus and the result was okayish. However, most of these medicines were not beneficial when tried with Covid-19 real patients. Thus, it is "often" not useful.

- As for Celebrex, the main evidence came from a Spanish study on the computer, not on humans, not even on animals or even in a laboratory. The computer has revealed that its mechanism of action may work with the virus. Only a small weak study states that it may have a "secondary" effect against the virus. Is that enough for us to take it? No.

- Clinical trials have already proven that Remdesivir can speed up the recovery period from fifteen to eleven (15-11) days, but does not reduce mortality rates. Thus, most likely, it is beneficial, unlike Avigan, which clinical trials are not in its favor so far.

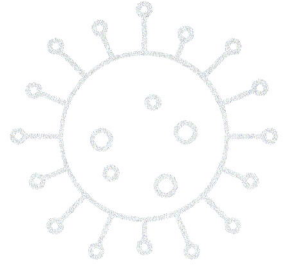

CHAPTER 25

ELI LILY'S GOOD NEW TREATMENT FOR HOME PATIENTS

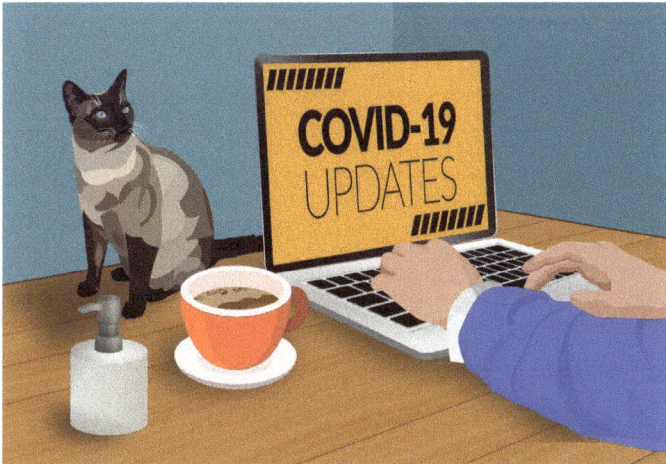

Eli Lilly[23] has announced good news, which we hope will finally prove credible. Eli Lilly is a well-known reputable American pharmaceutical company established 144 years ago with branches in 18 countries. It was a pioneer in spreading the polio vaccination and human insulin to treat diabetes. It is currently the first pharmaceutical company in the world in manufacturing psychiatric drugs. However, what was that good news? It has announced that its clinical trials of the drug LY-CoV555 have achieved very promising results regarding home treatment for mild and moderate cases.

The aim of this treatment is to stop the deterioration of the condition of the infected patients and reduce their need for hospitalization. It only works for the first three days following the emergence of the symptoms.

The treatment is a single injection of monoclonal antibodies[24] taken from the blood of a recovered patient and then processed in laboratories. It is similar to plasma treatment, but with an important essential difference,

---

23 Eli Lilly is an American pharmaceutical company headquartered in Indianapolis, Indiana, with offices in 18 countries. Its products are sold in approximately 125 countries.

24 Monoclonal antibodies are man-made proteins that act like natural antibodies in the immune system, but manufactured with big quantities in a single type to focus on a specific mission.

namely plasma contains many components, including those antibodies in small quantities and many other components that the patient does not need.

Here, the plasma is purified to obtain these antibodies specifically then engineered, processed, concentrated, and replicated in laboratories using very sophisticated techniques to reach a sufficient dose to kill millions of viruses efficiently.

The clinical trial began last June and included four hundred fifty-two (452) patients in two groups one of which received the antibodies while the other group received a placebo[25]. The results showed that the number of patients who needed hospitalization decreased by seventy-two percent (72%) after the injection and without any side effects. Most patients who needed hospitalization were elderly or obese, which indicates the priority for these groups of patients to receive treatment in case of infection.

The company tried three different doses of antibodies, and the best results were with the average dose, which

---

25 It is anything that seems to be a "real" medicine but it is not. It could be in any form. What all placebos have in common is that they do not contain an active ingredient meant to improve health.

significantly reduced the virus quantities eleven (11) days after the infection. This raised questions for some experts because the higher dose should have produced better results. Therefore, they advised not to exaggerate the importance of the new treatment until after the final results following trying it on other four hundred (400) patients and comparing it to another type of antibody named LY-CoV016. Other impartial experts considered the results and confirmed their promising credibility. On its part, the US Food and Drug Administration (FDA)[26] has authorized the continuation of experiments on the drug before its commercialization and approved it initially. The company is seeking to obtain additional approval for its use in emergencies until the experiments are completed.

An update as per the 14th of October 2020 news: The experiments for this new treatment were temporarily withheld due to safety concerns under investigation.

Ref rences 38 and 39

---

26 The Food and Drug administration is a US agency responsible for protecting the public health by ensuring the safety, efficacy, and security of human and veterinary drugs, biological products and medical devices.

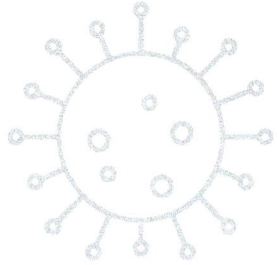

CHAPTER 26

CORONAVIRUS PREVENTION ADVICE AFTER RE-OPENING

Studies suggest Covid-19 transmission is much less likely in outdoor spaces than indoor settings

Researchers traced the contacts of 110 people with Covid-19, and recorded when the virus was passed on to a contact, split by whether or not the primary case had met people indoors

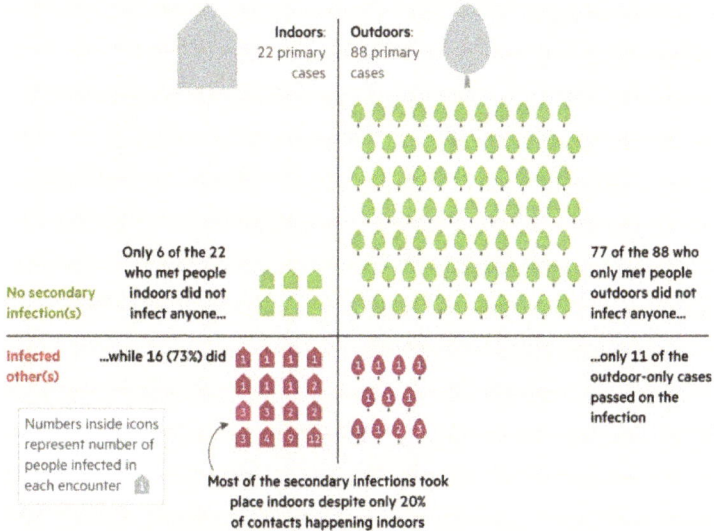

Indoors: 22 primary cases

Outdoors: 88 primary cases

No secondary infection(s)

Only 6 of the 22 who met people indoors did not infect anyone...

77 of the 88 who only met people outdoors did not infect anyone...

Infected other(s)

...while 16 (73%) did

...only 11 of the outdoor-only cases passed on the infection

Numbers inside icons represent number of people infected in each encounter

Most of the secondary infections took place indoors despite only 20% of contacts happening indoors

Source: Nishiura et al, Closed environments facilitate secondary transmission of coronavirus disease
© FT

In around 70% of cases, an infected person does not infect anyone else. In fact around 80% of new infections come from around 20% of cases

Share of index cases who go on to infect 0 more people, 1 more person, 2 more etc (%)

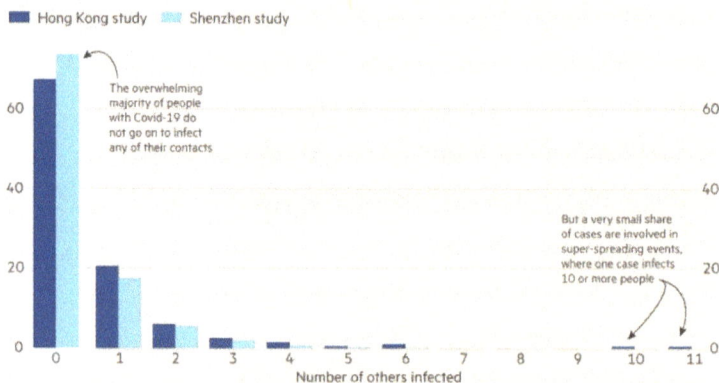

■ Hong Kong study ▨ Shenzhen study

The overwhelming majority of people with Covid-19 do not go on to infect any of their contacts

But a very small share of cases are involved in super-spreading events, where one case infects 10 or more people

Number of others infected

Adam et al. Clustering and superspreading potential of severe acute respiratory syndrome coronavirus 2 (SARS-CoV-2) infections in Hong Kong
Qifang et al. Epidemiology and transmission of COVID-19 in 391 cases and 1286 of their close contacts in Shenzhen, China: a retrospective cohort study
© FT

Coronavirus is more likely to spread in indoor settings where there is close and repeated personal contact

Share of people in each type of place who became infected after contact with an infected case (%)

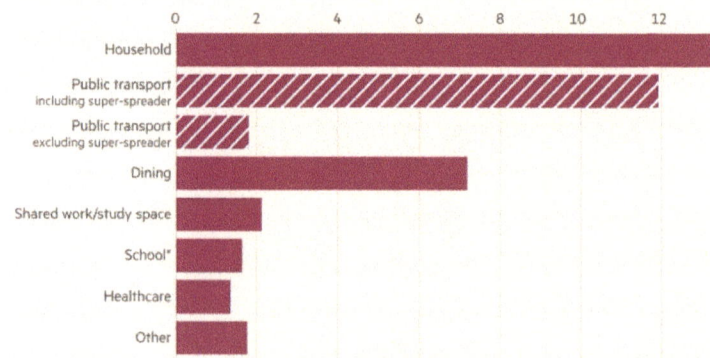

Household	
Public transport including super-spreader	
Public transport excluding super-spreader	
Dining	
Shared work/study space	
School*	
Healthcare	
Other	

Figures based on the tracing of 2,208 contacts of people infected with Covid-19
Data from Chen et al. Analysis of epidemiological characteristics of infection of close contacts of new coronavirus pneumonia in Ningbo.
*Danis et al. Cluster of coronavirus disease 2019 (Covid-19) in the French Alps, 2020
© FT

While the world is reopening, we have very important prevention advice in light of the latest scientific research on ways of Covid-19 spread.

1. About 90% of cases of infection occur in closed places. Do not be afraid of open spaces (streets, beaches, gardens, etc.) and be very careful in closed spaces, especially those crowded and poorly ventilated, (means of transportation, homes, offices, elevators, shops, cafes, restaurants, classrooms, lecture halls, etc.).

2. In a large research conducted on more than two thousand (2,000) cases, the houses were the first place of infection followed by the means of transportation, then the cafes and restaurants.

3. A comparison between buses and places of worship found that in a certain incident a group of people went to place of worship on a bus. The infection spread among thirty-seven of them thirty-five of whom on the bus and only two in the worship place.

4. In another incident, there was rehearsal for a concert in Washington attended by (60) sixty people fifty-two (52) of whom contracted the infection

from one asymptomatic person. This refutes the unfounded claim of the WHO, which backtracked on it later, that the asymptomatic patients do not transmit infection.

5. Infection from frequently touched surfaces is uncommon, but possible if you touch a surface freshly contaminated and then touch mouth or nose within minutes. This is more likely in common areas, such as elevator buttons, public bathroom faucets, doors knobs, computer keyboards, restaurant menus, banknotes, ATMs, stairwell, and escalator fences, shopping carts in the supermarket, etc. In this regard, shaking hands is like surfaces.

6. The period of contact is very important in transmitting infection: the longer the period, the greater the risk of infection, and vice versa .For example, if someone passes by you quickly, the chances of transmitting the infection to you is very limited. If you buy something from a store and go out in a few minutes, the chances of contracting the infection are low. If someone hangs out in the middle of the store while people are passing by her, the chances will increase.

7. The most common ways of infection are coughing and sneezing in the face of a person followed by talking closely with a person. If there is no coughing, sneezing, or talking from a close distance, the chances of infection are low and you will not contract the virus unless you remain close for an hour or more.

8. The effect of the mask decreases with the length of the mingling period. If there is direct chat with a person for more than five minutes, the effect of the mask will decrease.

9. The crowd has a very big impact in spreading the infection: parties, stuffed classes, weddings, small worship places, theaters, busy banks and government departments.

10. The conclusion is that we need to observe social distancing, wear masks, use hand sanitizers, mingle minimally when necessary, and go out in open spaces. We should know that the confined, crowded places with poor ventilation means infection by more than ninety percent (90%) and close to one hundred percent (100%) if you stay in the place for more than a few minutes.

☀ COVIDIOLA FOR TOMORROW

Flu vaccine is not to be missed during the winter season of the pandemic for the following reasons:

- The flu season was quite aggressive over the past couple of years. Possibly, this season will be the same.
- The symptoms of flu are very similar to those of covid, which will confuse both the doctor and the patient.
- You do not want to expose yourself to 2 types of serious infections within the same season, especially if your immunity is low or you suffer from any chronic disease, particularly heart and chest problems.
- In work places, schools, etc. if you get flu, you'll be treated unnecessarily as a suspected Covid with subsequent quarantine which may affect you financially.
- Flu infections with a second wave of Covid will double the burden on the healthcare system, adversely affecting the service, possibly leading to its collapse.

Reference 40

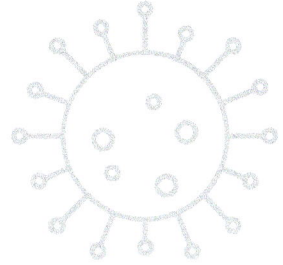

CHAPTER 27

CONGRATS FOR RECOVERY! ARE THERE LONG-TERM COMPLICATIONS?

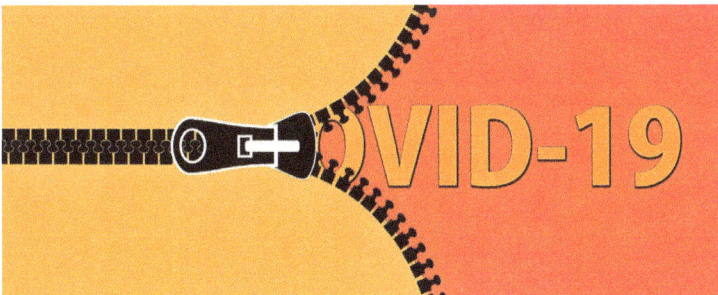

So far, the proven studies have indicated as follows:

1. During any severe infection, especially viral infection, complications may occur, including temporary hypercalcemia, temporary liver dysfunction, temporary leukopenia (low blood cell count) and thrombocytopenia (low platelet count), and temporary myositis (muscle inflammation).

2. If the condition of any patient with any disease generally deteriorates to the point of needing oxygen, ventilation, and intensive care, long-term complications may occur, such as lung damage, damage to brain and nerve cells, and impairment of the limbs, senses, or perception.

3. We now know that Covid-19 infection is one of the severest viruses known to humankind recently though the recovery percentage is about ninety-five percent (95%). As Covid-19 expanded to affect millions in few months despite different genetic and health backgrounds, and infection circumstances, we have seen an unprecedented diversity in the impact on the different body systems, be they the eyes, the nails, or the reproductive organs.

4. If a Covid-19 patient has become blind, for example, this should not be a cause for every other patient to panic. There are tens of millions of patients. If few lose their sight, the news will be on all the media. Even if 30-40 patients become blind, the odds are one in a million.

5. In sum, the vast majority of those recovering will have no complications, neither short nor long term.

The possibilities increase if the patient deteriorates to the point of needing intensive care.

6. What then should a recovered person do if they are afraid of complications? If there are no symptoms and tests during the illness did not reveal any complications, do not do anything at all. Forget Covid-19 and enjoy your life. If you feel any symptoms, or the tests during the illness revealed any defect (often temporary), follow up with your specialist physician until everything returns to normal, which may take up to several months.

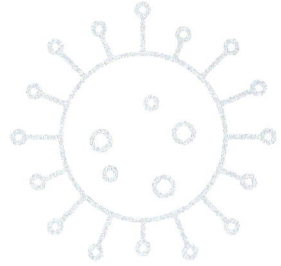

CHAPTER 28

HERD IMMUNITY: WHEN AND HOW?

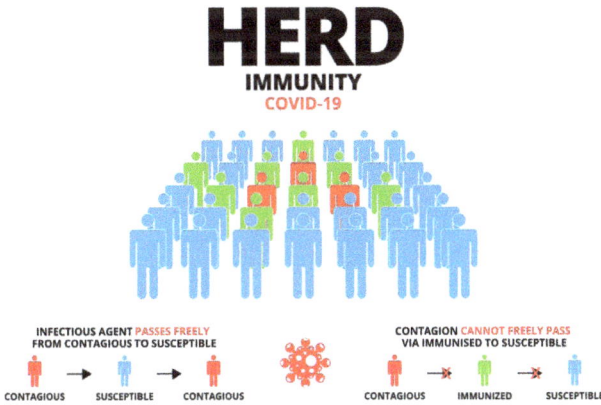

Scientifically, for herd immunity to materialize, at least sixty percent (60%) of the society must contract infection. When the British government tried to adopt herd immunity, the scientists warned against this because it simply meant an increase of two hundred and fifty thousand (250,000) deaths given that Britain's population is sixty-eight (68) million. Thus, Britain backtracked on this.

To know the extent of the virus spread in a society and if herd immunity is possible, we need a huge number of swabs, especially among the healthy people, to estimate whether those infected with the virus are close to sixty percent (60%) of the society. Let us get an idea of this hypothesis from the countries that conduct the largest number of swabs as of the summer of 2020:

- UAE: 317,000 swabs per million: 1.6% infected
- Denmark: 172,000 swabs per million: 1.3% infected
- Britain: 131,000 per million: 3.4% infected
- Russia: 126,000 per million: 3.5% infected
- Singapore: 116,000 per million: 6% infected
- Spain: 110,000 per million: 5.9% infected
- Portugal: 108,000 per million: 4.1% infected
- United States: 95,000 per million: 8% infected
- Kuwait: 87,000 per million: 12% infected
- Italy: 86,000: 4.8% infected

Therefore, infection rates in the world in general range from one to twelve percent (1%-12%) of members of the community. The majority is around five percent (5%). However, Qatar was an exception, where cases amount to twenty-seven (27%). It also has the lowest mortality rate (one per thousand). This may be due to the fact they are conducting swabs for a large number of healthy people as reflected in the staggering number of positive samples, i.e. ninety-three thousand (93,000) as of the summer of 2020, which was more than China, in a country with less than three million, and the limited number of deaths (because most people who test positive are healthy). We should not thus generalize Qatar's model due to its small size and population.

However, in any case, all countries of the world will take long to reach the sixty percent (60%) required for herd immunity. The pursuit of this in a country where, for example, the rate of infection is around five percent (5%) means that infection would multiply twelve times and so do the mortality rate.

In other words, herd immunity will not occur this year in any country. It may happen after a second and third wave, like the Spanish flu a century ago when herd immunity took place after three waves over three years. Otherwise, vaccination may emerge and relieve us from all of this if the virus does not mutate.

☼ **COVIDIOLA FOR TODAY**

Dutch-based group Glocalities has conducted a survey in Wuhan, where the pandemic started.

The survey included 2,022 Chinese. It has reported a significant shift of people attitude following the disaster. Among the main findings were:

- People placed much more emphasis on etiquette
- Individualistic behavior was unacceptable
- There was more desire for order and structure
- There was rising trust in education and institutions
- There was greater appreciation for those who contribute

References 41-43

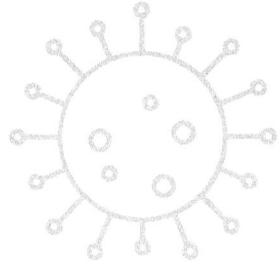

CHAPTER 29

HOW LONG WILL THESE MEASURES REMAIN? THAT IS THE QUESTION!

The answer to the above question requires a balance between two wings, that of controlling the pandemic and that of lockdown hazards, i.e. to reduce the economic, psychological, and social damage caused by the lockdown. The outlook is that the world countries, after a while, will begin to take different directions in terms of measures for several reasons:

First: The spread of the disease has entered different stages in each country. It is on the rise in some countries while others do not know if they will follow suit.

Second: In spite of spending the summer of 2020 co-living with the epidemic, we are still not certain of the effect of weather on the virus.

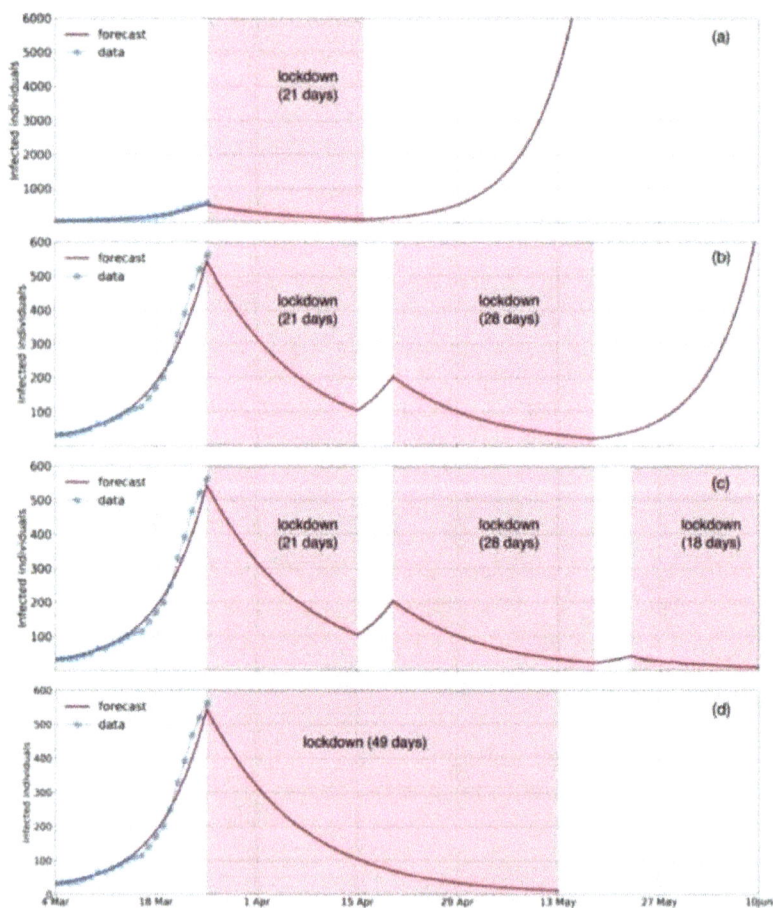

Figure 4. **Forecast of the COVID-19 epidemic in India with mitigatory social distancing.** Each of the four panels shows the variation in the number of infectives with lockdowns of various durations. The three-week lockdown starting 25 March does not prevent resurgence after its suspension as shown in panel (a). Neither does a further lockdown of 28 days spaced by a 5 day suspension, shown in panel (b). The protocols in panels (c) and (d), comprising of three lockdowns with 5 day relaxations and a single 49 day lockdown reduce case numbers below 10. This forecast is based on all cases being symptomatic so $\alpha = 1$. The fit parameter is $\beta = 0.0155$ and we set $\gamma = 1/7$.

Third: The attitudes of the heads of states differ. Rulers like Trump tend to favor the wing of minimizing the economic effects while other rulers care most about controlling the pandemic, whatever the economic effects may be, as is the case with most European countries.

Fourth: The conditions of the countries themselves differ. Some countries cannot afford a complete lockdown for a long time because, for example, they lack any plans and resources to support daily workers, farmers whose crops will be spoilt, etc.

Fifth: Some peoples are committed while others are not. This affects the way and extent of the disease spread, and hence the measures.

In terms of controlling the pandemic, a Cambridge study addressed the case of an Indian model (picture). It compared four types of preventive measures. In all four types, precautionary measures started after the cases reached five hundred (500).

i. In the first type, the measures lasted for three continuous weeks. The infections almost disappeared at the end of this period, but as soon as the measures stopped, the cases returned to five hundred within two weeks and then exploded. This type of measures is a failure.

2. In the second type, they did the same, but gave the people a break for five days followed by another lockdown for four weeks. The same result: as soon as they opened, the cases exploded. All they achieved was that they delayed the explosion for three months. This could be useful if you have an important change that will happen after the three months, such as vaccination or treatment, or you are sure, for example, that heat will eliminate the virus.

3. In the third type, they did the same, but after the second lockdown, people also took a 5-day break followed by 18-day lockdown. This time, they eliminated the virus.

4. In the fourth type, they had a lockdown for forty-nine (49) days without the 5-day break. They also eliminated the virus.

Accordingly, if we consider controlling the pandemic independent of economic, psychological, and social factors, the precautionary measures should last between one and a half months without interruption or two months and a half with short breaks. However, maybe every country will consider the numbers of the infected at every step.

If there are countries with too difficult conditions to bear this or if those in charge are more biased towards the economic side than controlling the pandemic, it is likely that the lockdown periods will be shorter than that.

In the end, every choice has a price. Every country should choose the option that suits it, the price it would pay, and the way it will do that.

⚛ COVIDIOLA FROM YESTERDAY

Following the middle ages black death plague epidemics in Europe, major developments for the better happened:

- Streets became wider
- Pavements were first introduced
- The job of street cleaners was created
- The sewage system was devised
- Wooden houses were abolished
- new agricultural hygienic methods were developed

What changes for the better you'd like to see following the current pandemic?

Reference 44

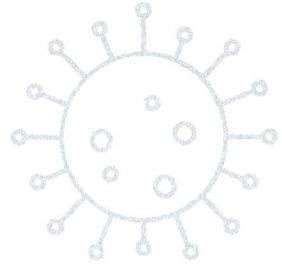

CHAPTER 30

REASONS FOR DELAYED VACCINATION

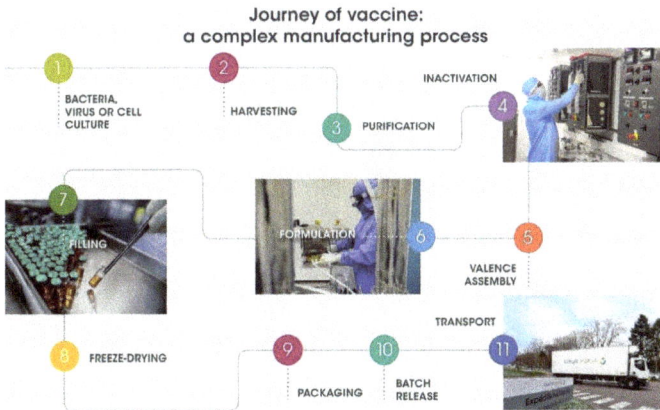

Journey of vaccine: a complex manufacturing process

Photo credit: Sanofi Vaccines Website

Some may ask why there will be no vaccination before 2021 even if the trials have recorded excellent, effective, and safe results today.

The answer is in the picture above. The eleven manufacturing steps need to be completed. In normal conditions, this would take between six months to three years. However, with this urgently needed vaccination, the manufacturers would speed up the steps, but we should not forget that the priority would be for the population of countries which produced the vaccination.

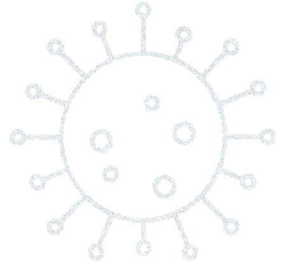

CHAPTER 31

THE PATIENT WHO STOPPED OXFORD VACCINATION TRIALS

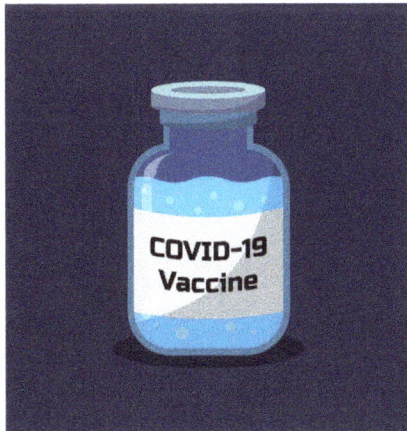

The Oxford-Astra Vaccination Team decided to resume vaccine trials after consulting with the responsible health authorities, thus reviving hope for approval being the vaccination closest to reaching the finish line in the clinical trials phase. There have been always broad hopes on this vaccine around the world to put an end to the nightmare of the pandemic.

The trials had stopped in September 2020 to ensure that the vaccination was safe enough after the vaccination research team found out that one of the volunteers developed transverse myelitis (TM)[27]. This caused panic because the disease, usually caused by a viral infection, rather rare and affects one out of every three hundred thousand (300,000) persons. Inflammation of the spinal cord leads to paralysis of the limbs and body organs below the level of inflammation. A third of patients recover completely after several months of treatment, a third becomes permanently paralyzed, and a third only partially heal.

However, the important question here is whether this infection was because of the vaccination or just an unfortunate coincidence given the vaccination was already tried on tens of thousands with no such adversity. Perhaps this person would have got the disease even if not injected with the vaccine. The answer to this question is almost impossible except through the continuation of

---

27 A rare neurological condition in which the spinal cord is inflamed. Transverse implies that the inflammation extends horizontally across the spinal cord.

the experiments and monitoring the rest of the people who take the vaccination. If the inflammation recurs to more than one person at a rate higher than the normal rate (1 per 300,000 people), there will be more doubts about the vaccination causing this dangerous side effect and this will reduce its chances compared to the rest of the vaccines that are currently in the trial race. However, if the number of people who receive the vaccination not developing transverse myelitis exceeds three hundred thousand people, then it is mostly just a misfortunate coincidence and this case will not form a potential risk of the vaccine.

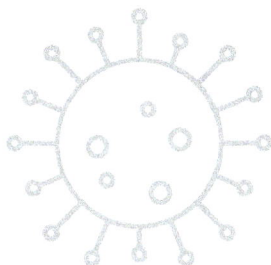

CHAPTER 32

WHEN WILL THE VACCINATION APPEAR? WHAT ABOUT THE PRICE?

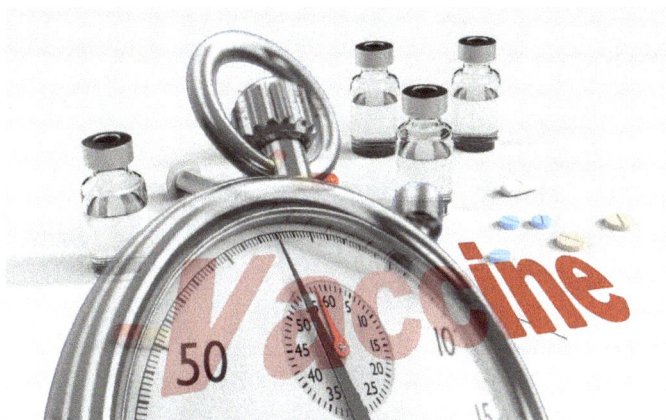

Leaving aside the Russian and the Chinese vaccinations due to the lack of transparency in the information published about them, the closest to coming to light are the three promising vaccines for Pfizer, Moderna, and Oxford AstraZeneca.

Several weeks ago, the AstraZeneca vaccination was the closest to reaching the finish line by ending the final phase of the trials in September 2020, but as discussed in the previous chapter an unfortunate event happened when one of the vaccinated patients developed transverse myelitis. Research is still ongoing to make sure that it was not a side effect of the vaccine.

Accordingly, the Oxford AstraZeneca vaccination fell to third place in terms of the priority to mass production.

The statements of Pfizer and Moderna officials about the readiness of their vaccinations mentioned the end of October and the beginning of November for release. Trump was more optimistic, as he stated during his "election propaganda" that the vaccination would be ready before mid-October.

Of course, this has not happened until the time of publication of this book in the second week of October 2020.

Nevertheless, apart from the commercial and political statements of the two companies and Trump's politics, the scientific opinion of vaccine and communicable disease experts in the United States confirms that the vaccination of most of the US population will not take place before mid-2021. Unfortunately, Adar Poonawalla, chief executive officer of Serum Institute of India (SII), the largest vaccine producer in the world, stated that the vaccination of the entire world population would not take place before 2024 at best. However, the good news is that the price of the vaccine will be very cheap, in the tune of US$3 dollars per dose.

☼ COVIDIOLA FROM YESTERDAY

Our human civilization learnt a lot through the mayhem of world wars:

Plastic surgeries, portable x rays, vaccinations against Typhoid and Tetanus, limbs prosthesis and cans for food preservation were all parented by world war 1.

The difficult supply situation during world war 2 has forced people for a healthier eating style. The atrocities lead by Hitler brought about the need for new definitions of democracy and the necessity of unified Europe with common interests and benefits. The British NHS (National Health Service), one of the world's greatest was also a child of world war2.

Do you expect anything good out of the current epidemic lessons?

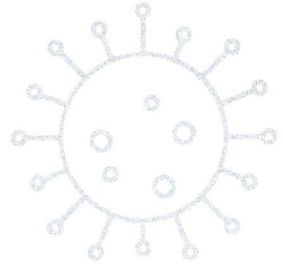

CHAPTER 33

THE PRICE OF THE PANDEMIC

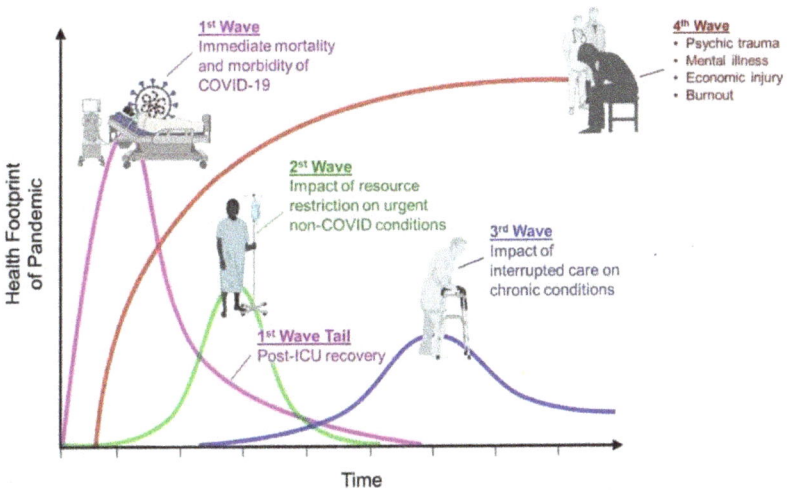

The current first wave: mortality and morbidity.

The second wave: the consumption of resources in dealing with the virus leads to the deterioration of other health emergencies, such as accidents, various causes of infection, heart attacks, stroke, etc.

The third wave: care for chronic diseases, such as cancer, diabetes, and kidney failure deteriorates.

Gradually, parallel to all this, the fourth wave resulting from economic, psychological, and nervous destruction and its consequences, including effects on peoples and countries, crime rates, and social and political unrest, will be escalating.

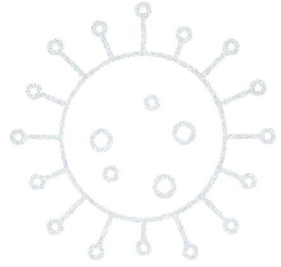

CHAPTER 34

SALUTE TO THE COUNTRY MOST SUCCESSFUL IN HANDLING THE CORONAVIRUS

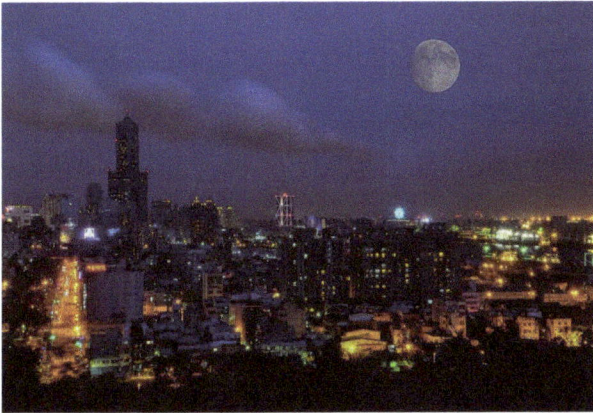

Just one country in the world has achieved great success in dealing with the coronavirus without imposing a lockdown or disrupting its economy.

Just one country in the world has flattened the curve before it rose in the first place though the cases appeared there at the beginning of the outbreak.

Just one country in the world preceded the WHO and its experts.

Just one country in the world preceded China in dealing with the pandemic.

Just one country did not receive assistance from the WHO because it is not a member.

This country did this simply because it had prepared one hundred and twenty-four (124) procedures signed by its President years ago. It only enforced these measures in one day.

This country began the one hundred and twenty-four (124) procedures on December 31, 2019 with the first unconfirmed news about the outbreak of the pandemic in China and weeks before the official announcement.

This country closed its borders with China and all surrounding countries at a time when the WHO was saying that there was no evidence that this virus was transmitted between people.

This country is only 180 km from China and thus classified as being one of the most countries the pandemic would devastate, but the exact opposite happened. In one day, the whole people wore masks, observed social distancing, and continued to work. In one day, they increased their production capacity of masks four times.

It was the first country to prevent the export of medical supplies. As soon as they controlled the pandemic, they donated ten million masks to the countries that stood by them.

It has wonderful advanced technology and a legendary network of information about the health conditions of every citizen and resident.

Since it is among the first-row democracies in the world, it took precautionary measures and wrote a heroic success story through democracy and transparency without oppression or suppression. The government used to call all those quarantined randomly to make sure they did not go out and gave each US$ 30 a day in order not to get out of isolation. In this way, citizens themselves were even keener than government to conduct tests and implement preventive precautions.

It was the first country in the world to invent rapid diagnosis and antibody tests for the virus and antibodies and to test all those arriving and departing in addition to all labor gatherings.

We should all salute Taiwan. At the time of publication of this book in October 2020, 8 months after the emergence of the epidemic in Taiwan, the total number of cases is only 518 cases, with 485 recoveries (94%), and only 7 deaths. The economy did not stop even for one day. We need all to salute Taiwan, that isolated country which was not helped by the international community to satisfy China and is not accepted as a member of World Health Organization to please China.

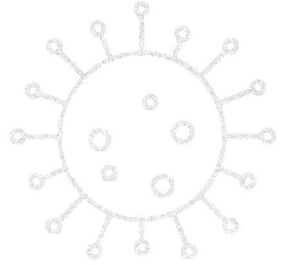

CHAPTER 35

THE SECOND WAVE.
WHAT TO EXPECT?

As evidenced by the attached pictures extracted from the statistical updates at the time of publication of this book; the first week of October 2020, the second wave of the pandemic has already started in the northern most countries of the north hemisphere.

From mid-September, there is a very significant surge of new cases which can not be missed, even by non-specialists.

This surge is not to be explained by relaxation of social distancing rules. It does not make sense that the relaxation has happened in multiple countries at the same exact point of time. It is also not explicable to be a false rise due to wider testing strategies, as there has been no recent change of these strategies at the same point by multiple countries.

It could be partially explicated by the resumption of school attendance after summer holidays. Yet, we have to consider that this is the exact point of time where the seasonal flu starts to surge every year. like flu virus, coronavirus and all the other respiratory viruses get much more active spread starting in the autumn and through the winter.

So, here we are. We are already on the ride of this curse for the next few months. Historically, the second wave of the Spanish flu was the worst of the three.

Daily New Cases in Canada

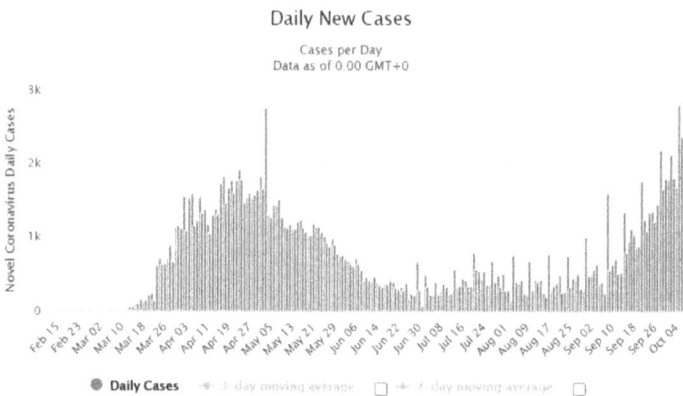

Daily New Cases

Cases per Day
Data as of 0.00 GMT+0

Daily New Cases in the Netherlands

Daily New Cases

Cases per Day
Data as of 0:00 GMT+0

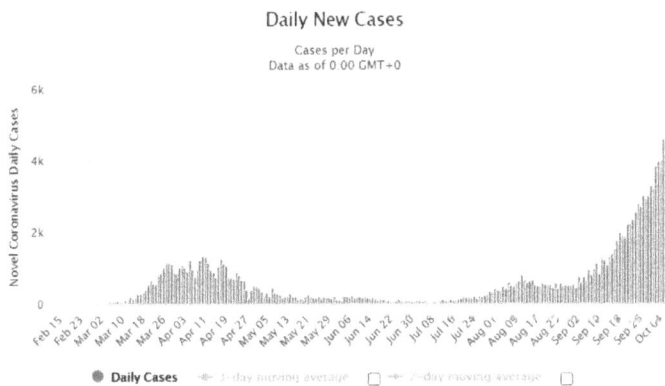

Daily New Cases in the United Kingdom

Daily New Cases

Cases per Day
Data as of 0:00 GMT+0

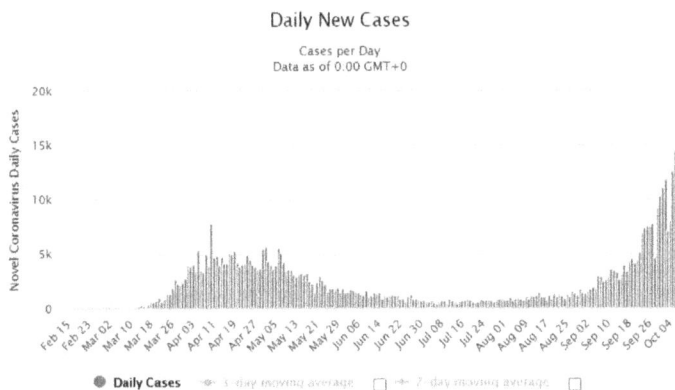

Daily New Cases in France

Daily New Cases

Cases per Day
Data as of 0:00 GMT+0

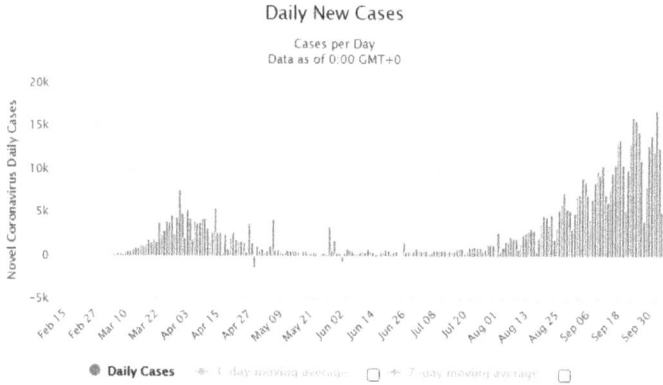

But wait, the scene is not that grim.

I have very good news to follow. Look at the next set of pictures.

Daily New Deaths in Canada

Daily Deaths

Deaths per Day
Data as of 0:00 GMT+8

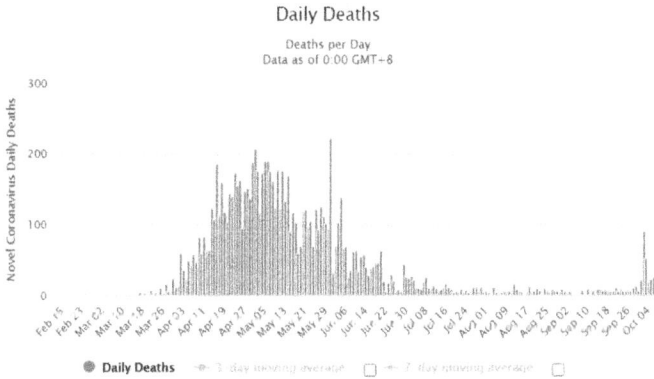

Daily New Deaths in the Netherlands

Daily Deaths

Deaths per Day
Data as of 0:00 GMT+8

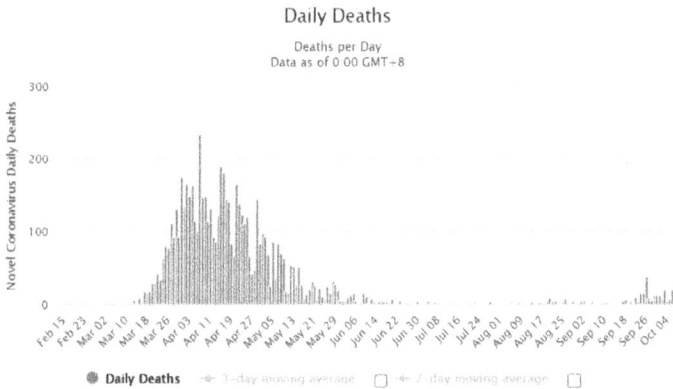

Daily New Deaths in the United Kingdom

Daily Deaths

Deaths per Day
Data as of 0.00 GMT−8

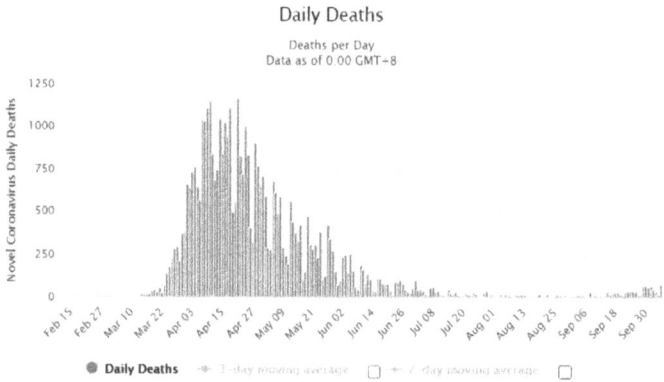

Daily New Deaths in France

Daily Deaths

Deaths per Day
Data as of 0.00 GMT−8

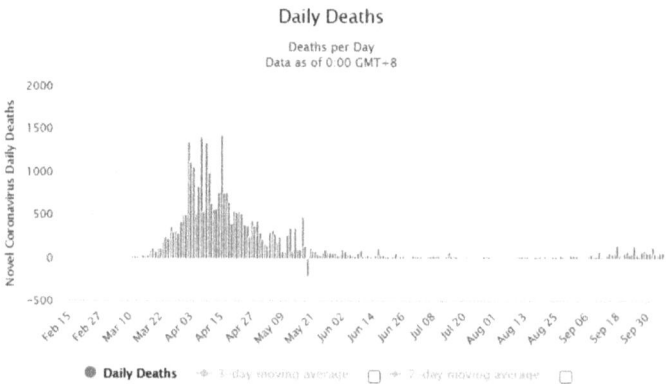

Although the numbers of daily cases of this second wave is much higher, there are very reassuring statistics about the death rate.

The new cases in the Netherlands are triple the peak of the first wave. In France it is more than double. In UK it is double. In Canada it is slightly higher.

But look at the death rates. They are very low, nothing to be compared to the first wave. We are dealing with less than 1% death rate. If you remember, the UK at one point had 16% death rate during the first wave. (See April statistics on the charts above). France even reached 18% death rate. The Netherlands had 13% death rate, and Canada had 10%.

Why are the death rates much less?
First, there is some strong evidence that the virus has become much less virulent.

Second: Health professionals are now much more experienced and organized in management of the cases.

Third: With much higher public awareness, people seek medical advice earlier and with observation of social distancing rules the gush of cases to hospitals is much slower.

Fourth: Governments have provided adequate supplies to healthcare systems, including; Critical care beds, wide range testing facilities, and equipment, especially ventilators. More professional staff were trained.

Fifth: Evidence based medicine has provided us with clearer guides in relation with what works and what causes harm in terms of medications.

What is the current concern?

My main concern at the moment is the simultaneous return of the seasonal flu with the second wave. We have already seen horrible flu seasons over the past 2 years, having hospitals and critical care units loaded with sick people. Fortunately, last year the Covid19 started at the end of the winter, so we did not encounter overlap of the 2 viruses. It will happen now.

Lockdown again??!!

Personally, I believe that the world can't afford another full universal lockdown. I will elaborate more on that within the next chapter. Probably, it is not of that great benefit as well from the pure epidemiological perspective, bearing in consideration the current lower mortality rate, the continued observation of social distancing and the wiser selective lockdown which can be implemented on specific areas and categories of the population, depending on the statistics and relative risks.

I expect and support dynamic selective temporary lockdowns as needed.

Hopefully, one or more of the vaccinations will get the final stamp soon and can achieve global distribution before the end of the spring.

Recommendations I suggest

- I advise every single person, starting from the age of 6 months to have the flu jab.
- Social distancing and wearing masks should be even more strict.
- Deployment of wider rapid testing for both flu and corona
- Unending the current governmental support to the healthcare system by funding and boosting more research, training, professionals' employment, supply of equipment, especially ventilators and critical care unit beds.
- Dynamic selective temporary lockdowns
- Shielding of high risk groups for 3 months

- Planning and funding the global distribution of one or more of the coronavirus vaccines as soon as they get the final stamp.
- Thinking out of the box in relation to decentralization of health services and the wide use of ambulatory units for testing, emergency treatment and respiratory support.

☀ COVIDIOLA FOR TOMORROW

During the first wave of the pandemic, it was found out that the death rate had been much better in countries with higher number of critical care beds and ventilators in relation to the population.

One of the key elements for victory over the second wave is to ensure the adequate supply of such facilities and equipment considering the simultaneous surge of seasonal flu cases.

References: 43, 45 & 46

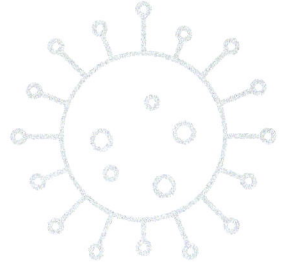

CHAPTER 36

THE PANDEMIC ECONOMY

Majority of countries on the brink of recession
Real GDP growth, Q1 2020

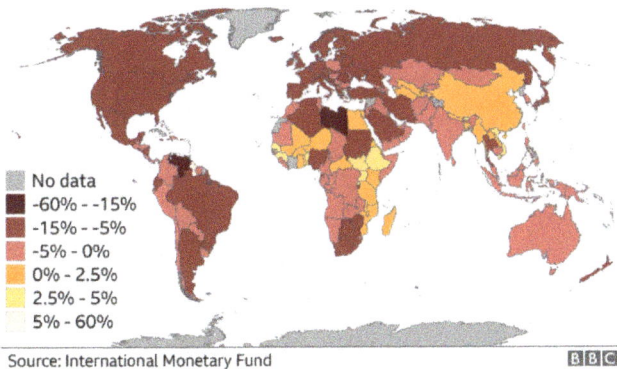

No data
-60% - -15%
-15% - -5%
-5% - 0%
0% - 2.5%
2.5% - 5%
5% - 60%

Source: International Monetary Fund

A detailed specialized economic analysis and discussion of the pandemic and its sequelae, including the lockdown are beyond the spectrum of this book. But, touching on this crucial perspective is indispensable. At the point of publication of this book, October 2020, more than 1 million people have already died by the viral infection. Deaths by the pandemic economic sequelae will follow. It will be difficult to count them accurately, due to complexity of the issue. Nevertheless, some experts estimate them to be more than the infectious deaths. Millions lost and will continue to lose their jobs, political and social unrest will have its victims. Suicides, homicides, and more. Disruption of logistics for the essentials, especially in poor countries will multiply the toll. Even within the healthcare sector itself, priorities have been shifted from other lethal illnesses like cancer, stroke, renal failure and disabilities for the sake of the coronavirus battle. Chapter 33 of this book has already touched on with an illustration on this matter.

It is not only about deaths, but also quality of life deprived from essentials of welfare.

All over history, epidemics have disrupted life, reforms, and progress of civilization. Yet, the current pandemic is unprecedented, considering the 21st century shape of life on this planet.

The figure shows the International Monetary Fund reflection of growth all over the world in the first quarter of 2020. This is not the lockdown effect. This is the pre-lockdown effect. Most countries of the world were already on the brink of recession. Needless to say what happened afterwards.

A research titled: "Global macroeconomic scenarios of the Covid-19 pandemic" published by the Australian National University expected that the world economy will suffer a loss of $17.3 trillion this year.

For example, in USA, the number of labor force participants not at work quadrupled from January 2020 to April of the same year. The number of people not in the labor force who want a job spiked by 4.5 million in April and has remained elevated. Small business revenue is down 20 percent from January 2020 till September 2020.

Nearly all sectors of business have been traumatized by varying extents. Some sectors may recover soon if a vaccine comes out in the near future. Sectors like travel, tourism and entertainment will struggle for years even if the epidemic ends tonight.

Some business went bankrupt as the damage was irreversible.

Governmental spending on combating the virus and compensations will never come back.

What we should do next will remain always a matter of balance between the direct saving of lives through the battle against the obvious infectious enemy and saving them indirectly through the long term war against the masked economic foe.

References: 47, 48

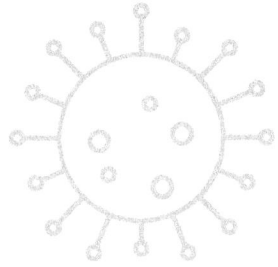

CHAPTER 37

WILL THE CORONAVIRUS TEACH US LESSONS IN JUSTICE AND WISE GOVERNANCE?

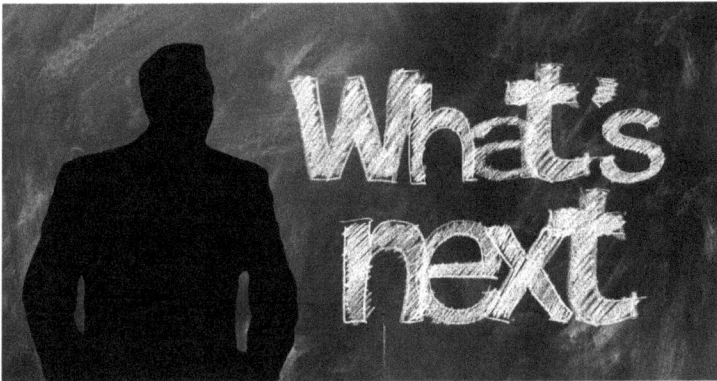

Placing too many workers in crowded housing leads to the closure of the factory and bankruptcy of its owner.

Crowding in public transportation spreads the virus, killing the owner of the luxurious car.

The house cleaner who lives in the slums transmits the disease to the elite he serves.

A waitress whose restaurant manager refuses to grant her a sick leave will infect the well-dressed clients.

Unhygienic practices in a random market in the Far East are destroying the lives of the celebrities of high-end societies in the far west.

The advocates of absolute personal freedoms are locked in their rooms due to the excessive personal freedoms of others they do not even know.

The rich man who evades taxes will not find a ventilator to save his life due to the state's inability to spend on healthcare.

A dictator ruler who spreads ignorance and backwardness among his people is not safe along with his family and entourage from death because of the practices of the citizens he governs .

A country that scatters money on arms deals and security fortifications has more deaths from the virus in a week than in a year of war or one hundred terrorist attacks.

Officials of a state that did not spend on training physicians, educating nurses, and providing them with a decent living, will not find someone to save their lives when it is not possible for them to be treated abroad.

The state that has spent on the tallest tower, the largest mosque, the largest church, and the widest bridge will spend exponentially on compensating construction companies that have gone bankrupt.

A country that lacks insurance, pension, and compensation laws will pay billions to save its society from political unrest, crimes, and chaos after the collapse of the economy and widespread unemployment.

The military ruler, who replaced freedoms with iron fist will not find commitment, discipline, or reform where the iron fist has no chance to succeed.

The superpower that supported tyranny in another country loses because of absence of transparency, false claims, misleading figures, and twisting of facts inherent in the dictatorial propaganda.

Will Professor Coronavirus then teach the world much needed lessons in justice, human conscience and wise governance?

☀ COVIDIOLA FOR TOMORROW

In April 2020, a survey conducted by "you gov UK" and the Royal agricultural society which included 4343 subjects has found out that 91% of people do not want life in the post-covid era to go back to how it was before the pandemic. They said that the air is now cleaner due to closure of factories, families are getting closer, and there is more sense of community. The wild life is being restored away from cruel human interference. The survey contributors started now to save more money, cook at home and stopped buying junk.

"It shows a real appetite for change and to learn from the crisis" said professor Tom Mcmillan from the Royal Agricultural Society

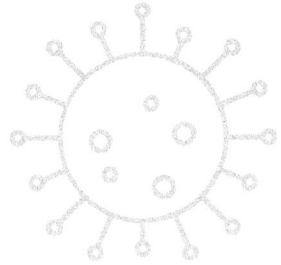

THE POST-COVID ERA

Covid winners

Like all other crises throughout history, it is not a season of losses for everybody. There are always chances, gains and benefits for some. Jeff Bezos, the CEO of Amazon nearly doubled his gigantic wealth just in 8 months, expanding it by 87 billion $ more. All online businesses have flourished. Visa, Pfizer, Microsoft and others have made huge profits. The global hand sanitizer market had 600% growth, reaching 1.87 billion $. The wealthiest 500 billionaires have augmented their worth by 813 billion $.

In the eyes of conspiracy theorists, all of those have contrived, manufacturing the pandemic to win such gains. Trumpians might think differently, but still within the conspiracy zone. Well, it must be the democrats and Chinese who made it up to interpose America's march to be great again before the next elections. The same goes for populists following Bolsonaro in Brazil or Sisi in Egypt. Evil enemies of the state are trying to destroy it.

Elements for excellence

But this is not the case indeed. If a volcano erupts tomorrow, these winners will still make immense profits and America's presumed march will be suspended. If aliens invade the earth, the same will happen. There is not necessarily a causal relationship between the winners and losers of any event.

Rationally thinking, the winners made such returns due to 3 elements: Readiness, flexibility and creativity. You can add to them perseverance at personal level . "Half the genius is perseverance" as once quoted from Naguib Mahfouz, the famous Egyptian literature Nobel laureate.

Having these elements will massively boost your position whatever the situation you are in.

The creativity has been there all the time at Amazon, Microsoft, Facebook, google, You tube. The founders just cemented it with the other elements.

At governmental level, look at the example mentioned in chapter 34 of this book, the most successful country during the pandemic, which has not received any support from WHO or the international community: Taiwan. Years before the pandemic they had 124 procedures to face such situation in case it happens, already approved by the president (readiness). They implemented them at once and kept the economy going (flexibility).

An unfair world

The billionaires who gained from the pandemic just had enough readiness and flexibility to shift their businesses from whatever sector they were investing in to health-care and Technology.

But how can the tea plantation workers in India be that ready and flexible after their only source of income was suspended due to quarantine?

How can the 2 million textile workers in Bangladesh be ready and flexible to make a living after cancelling orders and shutting down their factories?

What about waiters in restaurants and airlines hosts who were fired?

Unfortunately, there are no equal opportunities in this world. Majorly, it is out of your hands.

If you dig at Bezos' example. He did not do it from scratch. He started with 300,000 $ gift from his rich adoptive father (His biological father was an ordinary bike shop owner). Then, money makes money (Only if you have flexibility, creativity, and perseverance). So, you can add "Good luck" on top of the other elements.

There is nothing wrong with huge businesses expanding their profits as long as they are from legal and ethical sources. On the contrary, such businesses open opportunities for many and help the world in various ways: They are employing hundreds of thousands, making our lives easier and more enjoyable. Bill Gates is leading the vaccination race for Covid19 in addition to vaccination for Malaria and HIV. Elon Musk will provide the cheapest internet ever. Etsy[28] helped ordinary people to sell hundreds of millions of home- made face masks. You tube and Tiktok are great to showcase talents of the youth next door. At personal level, I wouldn't have published this book without Amazon/Kindle direct publishing.

---

28 An American e-commerce website focused on handmade or vintage items and craft supplies

Yet, all of this is very trivial looking at the majority who struggle for living. Half of the world population live on less than 6 $/day. Billions do not have access to proper healthcare, sanitation, accommodation and education.

I just touched on the issue of the top 500 billionaires in the world with many of them shifting their businesses during the pandemic to healthcare.

So, what are they selling?
Answer: Medical equipment to face the pandemic crisis.

To whom are they selling the equipment?
Answer: To governments.

From where is the government getting the money?
Answer: From public spending

So, the poor African lady who got Covid19 because of her poor living and working conditions won't get any treatment until her government uses the lady's own pennies to buy a ventilator from a multi-billionaire so that he can add a million more to his 5 billion. Does this sound right? Does it sound fair?

Time for change

Like the post-plague era, post-world war 1 era, and post-world war 2 era, the post-Covid era is time for change.

There will be definitely changes affecting all aspects of life; the "new normal" as they call it.

- If we are blessed with some good luck, are we ready for it?
- Are we being flexible?
- Are we creative enough?
- Are we going to persevere?
- Is your business/job able to survive and flourish online only?
- Do your work proceedings fit with people's panic from the next epidemic?
- Do you have adequate creativity to innovate a benefit from the global changes?
- Are you equipped with qualifications to be indispensable when 50% of the taskforce are fired?

At state and world levels, the top leaders, elite and moguls of power and money will try their best to own the change as usual. They have the highest chances to twist it and keep the current unfair world running "business as usual". Many of us were suffering in the pre-Covid era and many were keen to change the pre-Covid world for the better, a world of polarization, racism, environmental pollution, inequality, fake democracies, materialism, conflicts, militarization, corruption and spending on arms, security and propaganda rather than education, healthcare and scientific research. What is good in our eyes is bad for their pockets.

The Covid era is a fertile soil for conspiracy theorists, Trumpians and opportunistic earners. But, the post-Covid era can be a chance of good luck for reformists, only if they are ready, flexible, creative and persevere. Otherwise, we'll have to wait for the next disaster.

REFERENCES AND SOURCES

1. Strains of coronavirus—WebMD website

2. Human coronaviruses—CDC website

3. SARS—WHO website

4. MERS—WHO website

5. "The site of origin of the 1918 influenza pandemic and its public health implications". Journal of Translational Medicine. 2 (1): John Barry—Jan 2004

6. Just how contagious is COVID-19? This chart puts it in perspective—Matthew Francis—Popular science—February 2020

7. Large SARS-CoV-2 Outbreak Caused by Asymptomatic Traveler, China—Emerging infectious diseases—Jingtao Liu et al—June 2020

8. Health24 website: Yes, there is a 'right way' to cough and here's how—June 2019

9. Health24 website: How far can a cough travel?—December 2017

10. CDC website: Handwashing, when and how?

11. Why outbreaks like coronavirus spread exponentially, and how to "flatten the curve"?—The Washington Post—Harry Stevens—March 2020

12. The proximal origin of SARS-CoV-2—Kristian Andersen et al—Nature—March 2020

13. Absence of Apparent Transmission of SARS-CoV-2 from Two Stylists After Exposure at a Hair Salon with a Universal Face Covering Policy—Springfield, Missouri, May 2020—Joshua Hendrix et al—CDC website

14. N95 Respirators, Surgical Masks, and Face Masks—FDA

15. COVID-19: How much protection do face masks offer?—Mayo clinic

16. Understanding the Difference Between a Surgical Mask and N95 Respirator—JEMS—Daniel Berger- September 2020

17. Researchers created a test to determine which masks are the least effective—Alaa Elassar—CNN—August 2020

18. Oxford COVID-19 Evidence Service

19. The Incubation Period of Coronavirus Disease 2019 (COVID-19) From Publicly Reported Confirmed Cases: Estimation and Application—Lauer et al—Ann Internal Medicine—March 2020

20. Impact of non-pharmaceutical interventions (NPIs) to reduce COVID-19 mortality and healthcare demand—Ferguson et al—Imperial College response team—March 2020

21. Viral dynamics in mild and severe cases of COVID-19—Yang Liu et al—The Lancet—March 2020

22. Information for Pediatric Healthcare Providers—CDC—August 2020

23. COVID-19 (coronavirus) in babies and children—Mayo clinic

24. COVID-19 and Multi-System Inflammatory Syndrome in Children—Healthy children website

25. Children and COVID-19: State-Level Data Report—American Academy of Pediatrics—September 2020

26. COVID-19 in children and young people—Snape & Viner—Science—September 2020

27. Child deaths tied to covid-19 remain remarkably low eight months into U.S. pandemic—Lenny Bernstein—The Washington Post—September 2020

28. COVID-19 & Children Rapid Research Response UNICEF

29. Chinese attitudes shift as a result of coronavirus: survey—Luke Baker—Reuters—March 2020

30. Interpreting a Covid-19 test result—Jessica Watson et al—BMJ

31. Global partnership to make available 120 million affordable, quality COVID-19 rapid tests for low- and middle-income countries—WHO website—September 2020

32. Radiation risk from medical imaging (Harvard Health publishing)—January 2020

33. What are the Radiation Risks from CT?—FDA

34. Dexamethasone in Hospitalized Patients with Covid-19—Preliminary Report—The RECOVERY Collaborative Group—The New England Journal of Medicine—July 2020

35. COVID-19: Full Results of Dexamethasone Trial Confirm Benefits—Peter Russell—Medsccape—July 2020

36. Coronavirus breakthrough: dexamethasone is first drug shown to save lives—Heidi Ledford—Nature—June 2020

37. Coronavirus: Protein treatment trial 'a breakthrough'—Justin Rowlatt—BBC, July 2020

38. Antibody Therapy May Lower COVID Hospitalizations: Eli Lilly—Medical dialogues—September 2020

39. Eli Lilly reports promising first results for an antibody against COVID-19—Meredith Wadman—Science- September 2020

40. How to avoid the virus as the world reopens—Peel & Burn-Murdoch—Financial Times—June 2020

41. COVID-19 herd immunity: where are we?—Fontanet & Cochemez—Nature reviews: Immunology—September 2020

42. HERD immunity from Covid-19—What does it mean?—Narayana Health- June 2020

43. Worldometer website—Coronavirus updates

44. Age-structured impact of social distancing on the COVID-19 epidemic in India—Singh & Adhikari—Cornell University—March 2020

45. Coronavirus could be getting WEAKER, experts believe as infections rise but deaths remain low—The Sun—September 2020

46. Coronavirus is getting weaker, could disappear without vaccine—Boston news—June 2020

47. Covid-19 may cost global economy $35.3 trillion by 2025—Business—The National, UAE—Deepthi Nair—August 2020

48. Ten Facts about COVID-19 and the U.S. Economy—Lauren Bauer et al—Brookings institution, Washington—September 2020